Gross Anatomy Workbook

Gross Anatomy Workbook

THIRD EDITION

Achleshwar Gandotra
MBBS, Dip Ortho, MS Anatomy
Professor and Head
Department of Anatomy
Smt. BK Shah Medical Institute and Research Centre
Sumandeep Vidyapeeth
Vadodara, Gujarat, India

JAYPEE

JAYPEE BROTHERS MEDICAL PUBLISHERS
The Health Sciences Publisher
New Delhi | London | Panama

Jaypee Brothers Medical Publishers (P) Ltd

Headquarters

Jaypee Brothers Medical Publishers (P) Ltd
4838/24, Ansari Road, Daryaganj
New Delhi 110 002, India
Phone: +91-11-43574357
Fax: +91-11-43574314
Email: jaypee@jaypeebrothers.com

Overseas Offices

J.P. Medical Ltd
83 Victoria Street, London
SW1H 0HW (UK)
Phone: +44 20 3170 8910
Fax: +44 (0)20 3008 6180
Email: info@jpmedpub.com

Jaypee-Highlights Medical Publishers Inc
City of Knowledge, Bld. 235, 2nd Floor, Clayton
Panama City, Panama
Phone: +1 507-301-0496
Fax: +1 507-301-0499
Email: cservice@jphmedical.com

Jaypee Brothers Medical Publishers (P) Ltd
17/1-B Babar Road, Block-B, Shyamoli
Mohammadpur, Dhaka-1207
Bangladesh
Mobile: +08801912003485
Email: jaypeedhaka@gmail.com

Jaypee Brothers Medical Publishers (P) Ltd
Bhotahity, Kathmandu, Nepal
Phone +977-9741283608
Email: kathmandu@jaypeebrothers.com

Website: www.jaypeebrothers.com
Website: www.jaypeedigital.com

Gross Anatomy Workbook

First Edition: 2000

Second Edition: 2006

Third Edition: **2019**

ISBN 978-93-5270-500-9

Printed at: Paras Offset Pvt. Ltd., New Delhi

Dedicated to

The Students and Teachers of Anatomy;
Both Present and Past

PREFACE TO THE THIRD EDITION

In the recent past, textbook concept has changed to illustrative texts for better conceptualization of the subject. Keeping this in mind, in this edition, I have tried to make the illustrations more informative by adding relevant text. Some of the redundant diagrams have been deleted and some illustrations in the area of neuroanatomy is not provided with any text as they are self-explanatory.

I am sure this innovation would be liked by the students and faculties alike.

Achleshwar Gandotra

PREFACE TO THE FIRST EDITION

Anatomy has long been associated with a good working knowledge of drawing. A good hand at drawing is considered to be a prerequisite for the medical students and teachers alike. The drawing skill is an important factor in the medical education.

In many institutions in our country, it is mandatory for the medical students to complete Anatomical Record Journal. Most of the students find it an extra labor and sometimes a difficult job. I have the experience of the students finding it a monotonous exercise because it does not improve the drawing capability of the students and is time consuming. Since the time alloted to the first year MBBS has been truncated to just one year, so the time saving on the part of students is of prime importance.

Keeping these facts in view, I have for the first time, endeavored to produce the present *Gross Anatomy Workbook*. This workbook presents partially drawn and fully labeled diagrams. Meticulous care has been taken to incorporate only those diagrams which are relevant to the students from the examination point of view. A student is supposed to complete the diagrams and color them as per the standard norms of Anatomy. As a result, the students will have a colored atlas in hand. This entire exercise ensures that the student automatically will revise Anatomy, once he or she completes the workbook.

Therefore, I sincerely hope that the medical students would derive maximum mileage from this work.

I offer my apologies to the students and the teachers alike for the mistakes, if any, in drawing and labeling, despite meticulous proofreading.

At the end, I would like to offer my heartfelt gratitude to Dr ML Jain, Professor and Head, Department of Anatomy, Surat, for giving me the idea to produce this work. Thanks are due to the entire teaching staff of Anatomy, especially Dr CD Mehta (Associate Professor), Dr (Mrs) SS Bhagwat (Associate Professor), Mrs KB Vasu (Assistant Professor), Dr BB Gosai (Assistant Professor), all of Anatomy Department, Surat, and Dr BJ Gohil (Associate Professor), Anatomy Department, BJ Medical College, Ahmedabad, who gave their valuable suggestions and guided me during the making of this workbook.

Last but not least, I would like to thank my wife and children who showed great patience with me and stood by my side during the production of this work.

Achleshwar Gandotra

ACKNOWLEDGMENTS

The third edition of *Gross Anatomy Workbook* is a collective effort on the part of my colleagues who provided valuable suggestions, my students who prompted me to pen down salient features of the illustrations to help them in examinations and the publisher, Jaypee Brothers Medical Publishers (P) Ltd, New Delhi, India, who continuously prodded me to revise the book.

I sincerely thank:

Dr ML Jain—Formerly Head of the Anatomy Department, Govt. Medical College, Surat, Gujarat, India.

Dr CD Mehta—Formerly Head of the Anatomy Department, Govt. Medical College, Surat, Gujarat, India.

Dr (Mrs) Putul Banerjee—Formerly Head of the Anatomy Department, Smt. BK Shah Medical Institute and Research Centre, Surat, Gujarat, India.

Mr IN Wani—Assistant Professor, Department of Anatomy, Smt. BK Shah Medical Institute and Research Centre, Sumandeep Vidyapeeth, Gujarat, India.

Dr Manoj Kulkarni—Professor, Department of Anatomy, Smt. BK Shah Medical Institute and Research Centre, Sumandeep Vidyapeeth, Gujarat, for critically analyzing the text.

CONTENTS

PLATE 1

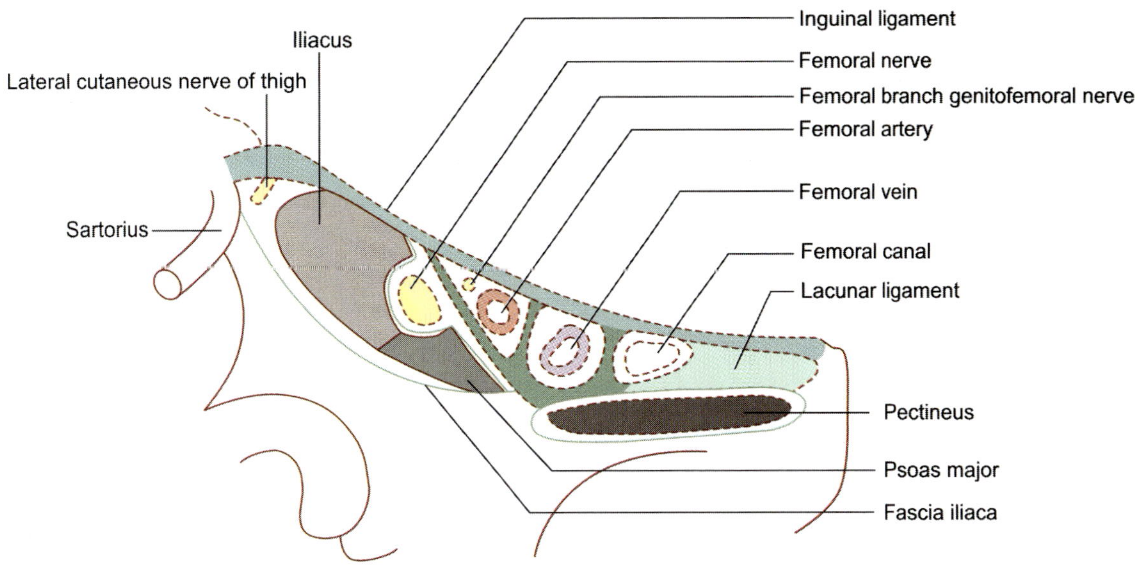

Figure 1.1: Structures passing under inguinal ligament

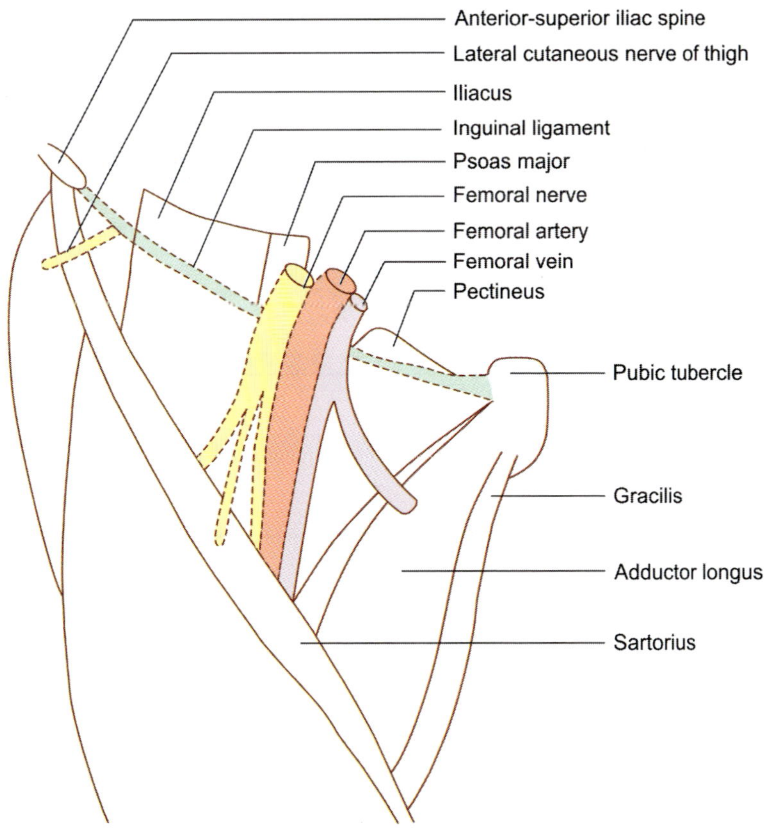

Figure 1.2: Femoral triangle

PLATE 2

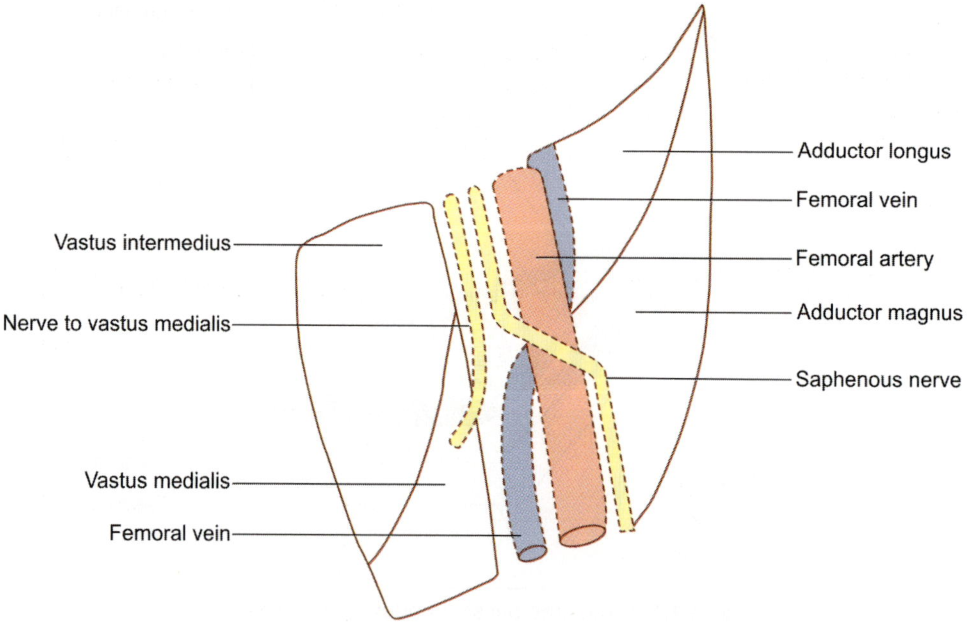

Figure 1.3: Adductor canal

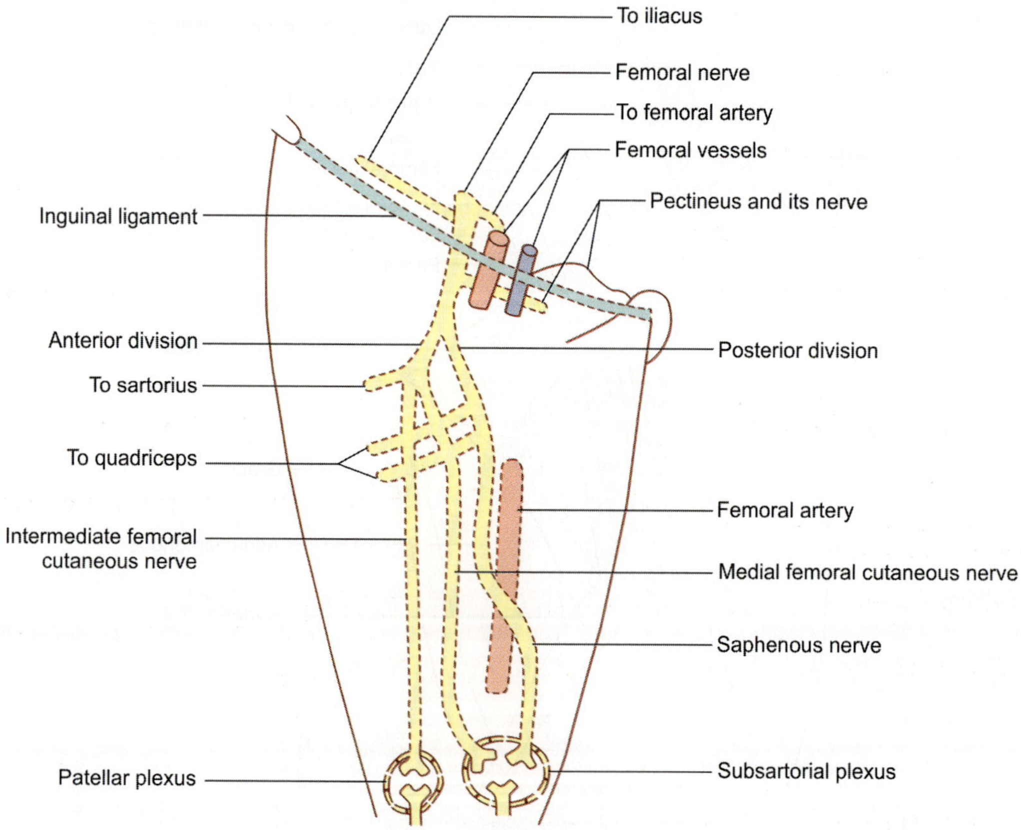

Figure 1.4: Femoral nerve

PLATE 3

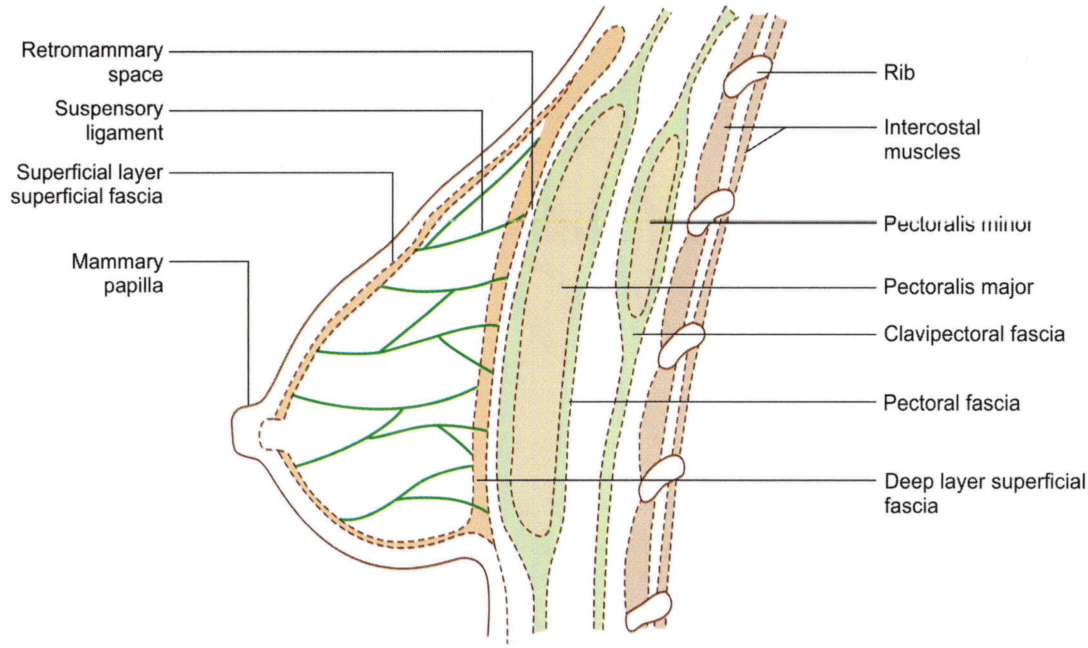

Figure 2.1: Mammary gland—relations

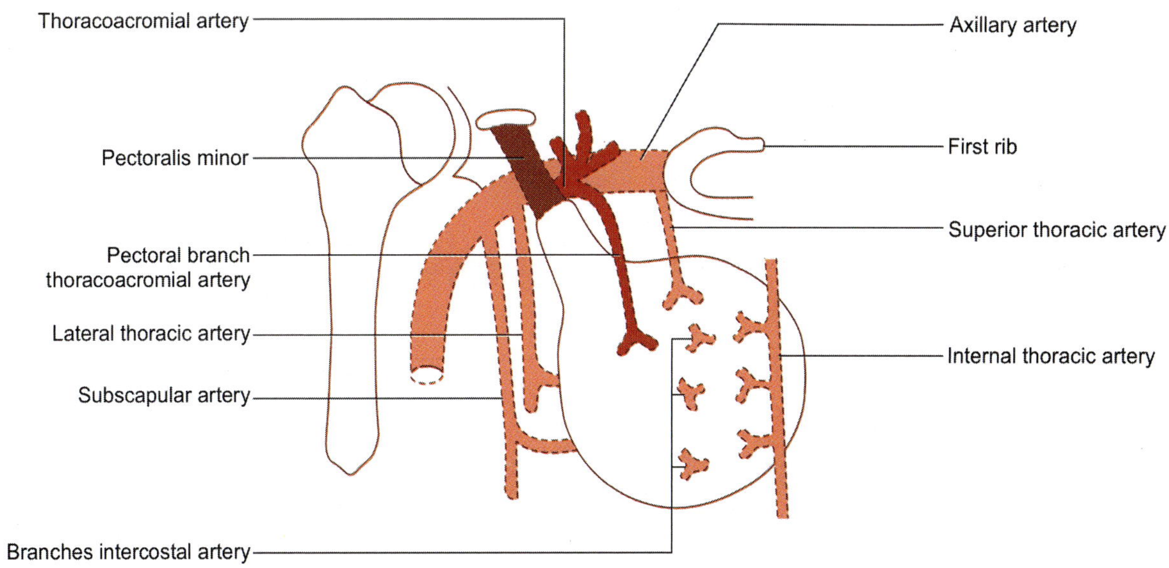

Figure 2.2: Mammary gland—blood supply

PLATE 4

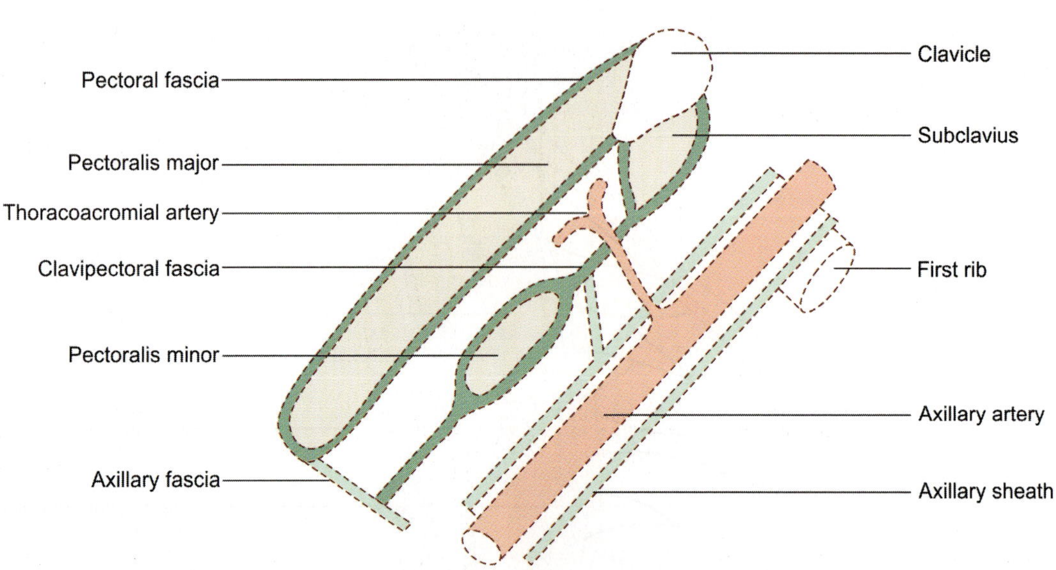

Figure 2.3: Clavipectoral fascia

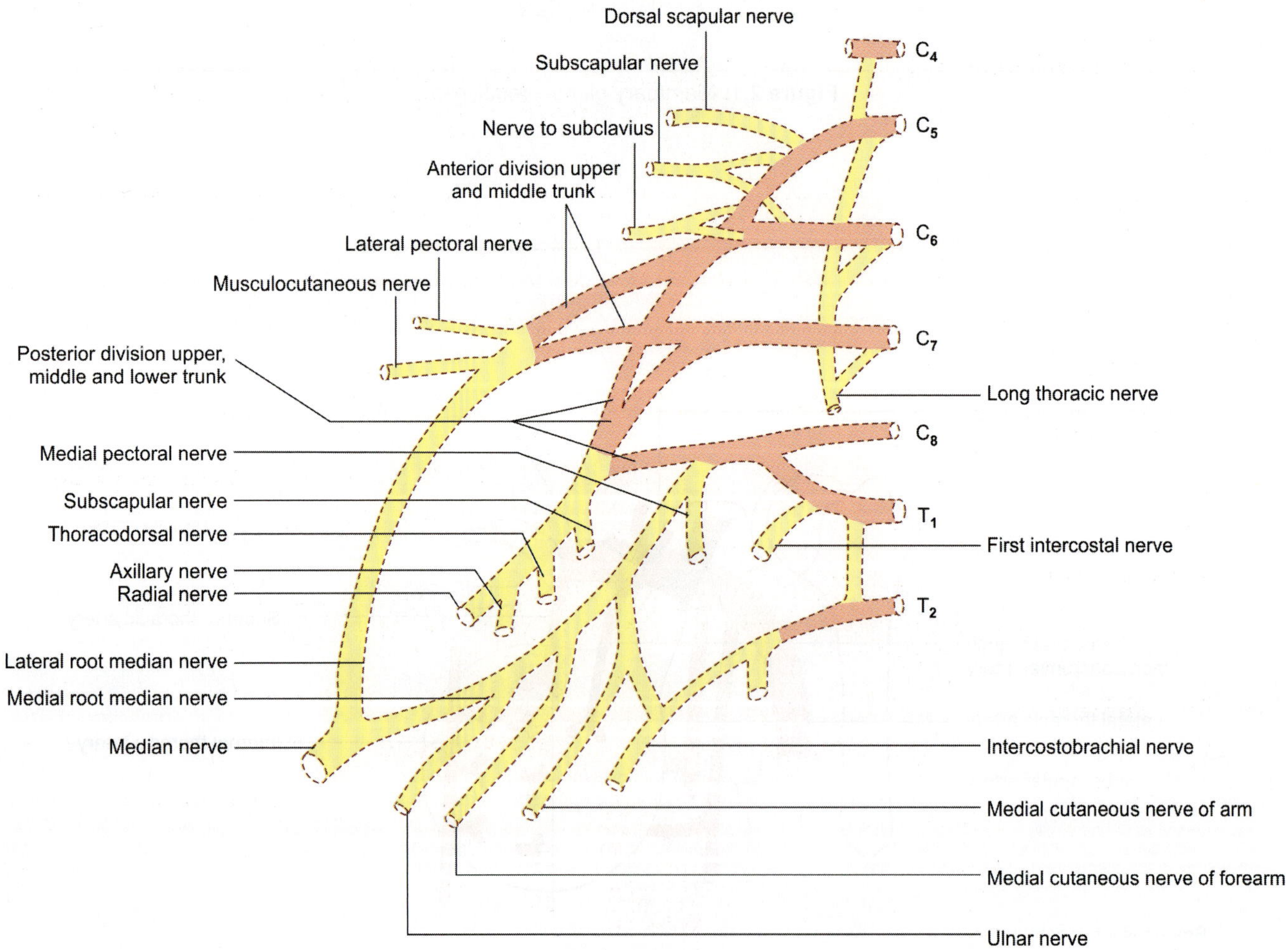

Figure 2.4: Brachial plexus

PLATE 5

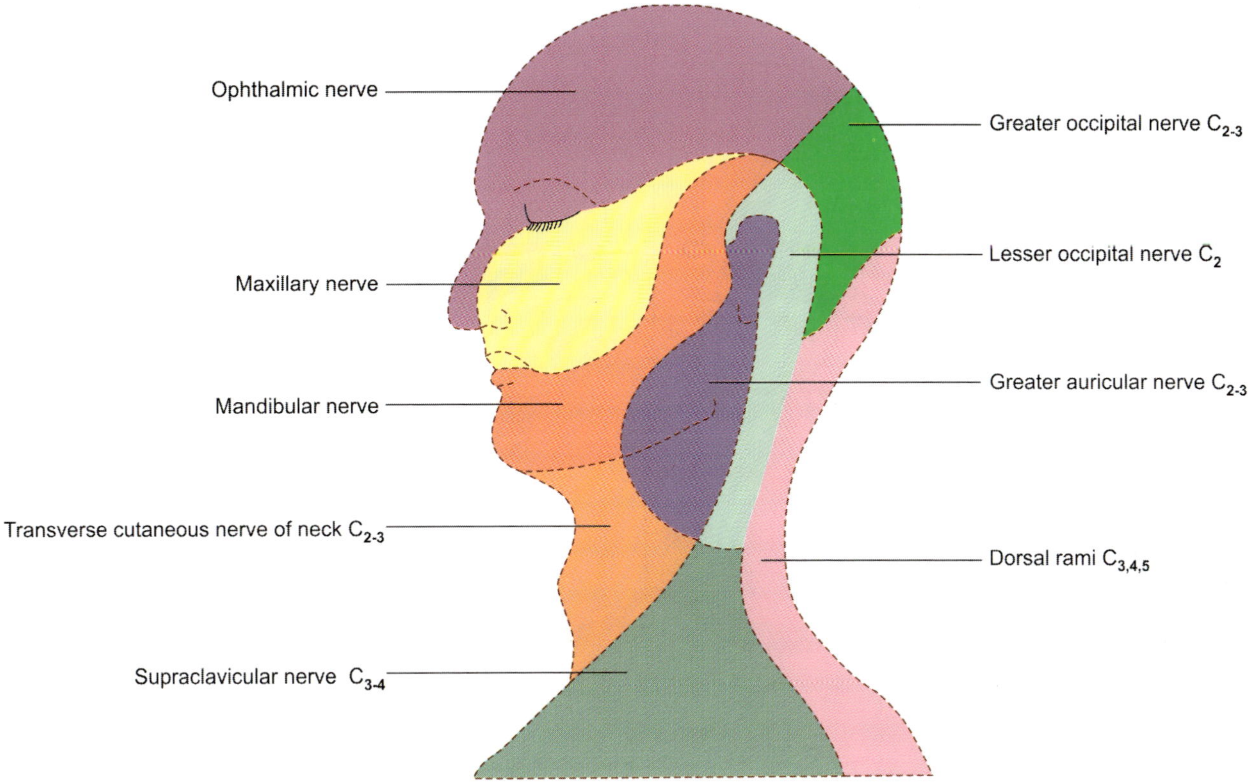

Figure 3.1: Dermatomes

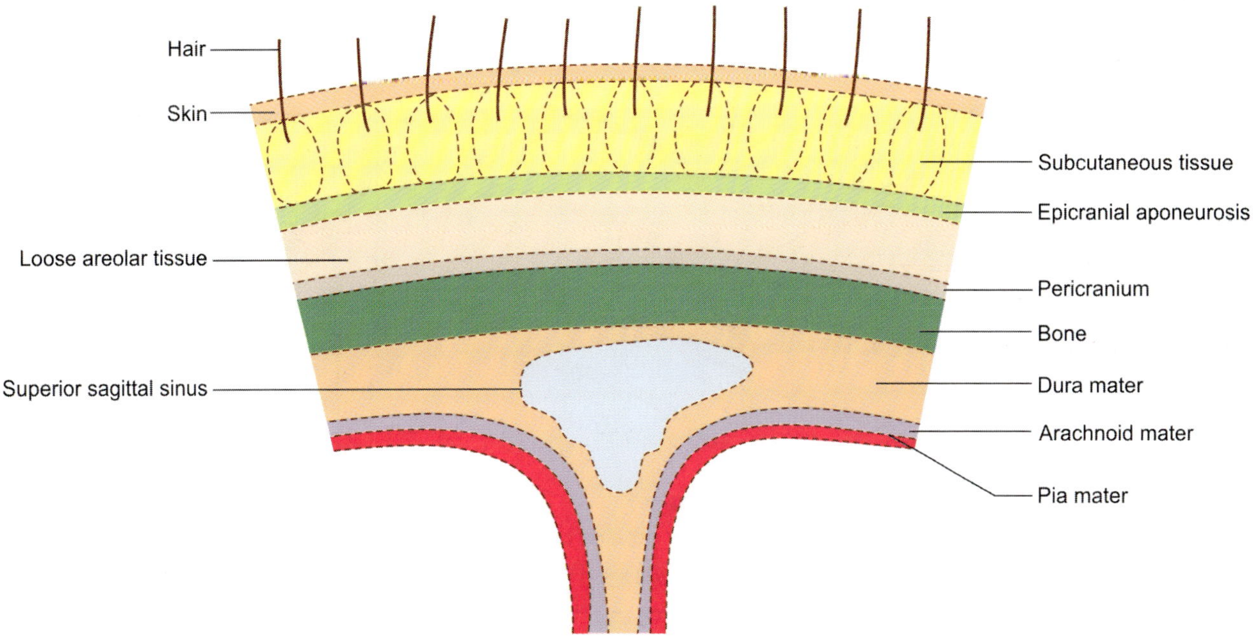

Figure 3.2: Layers of scalp

PLATE 6

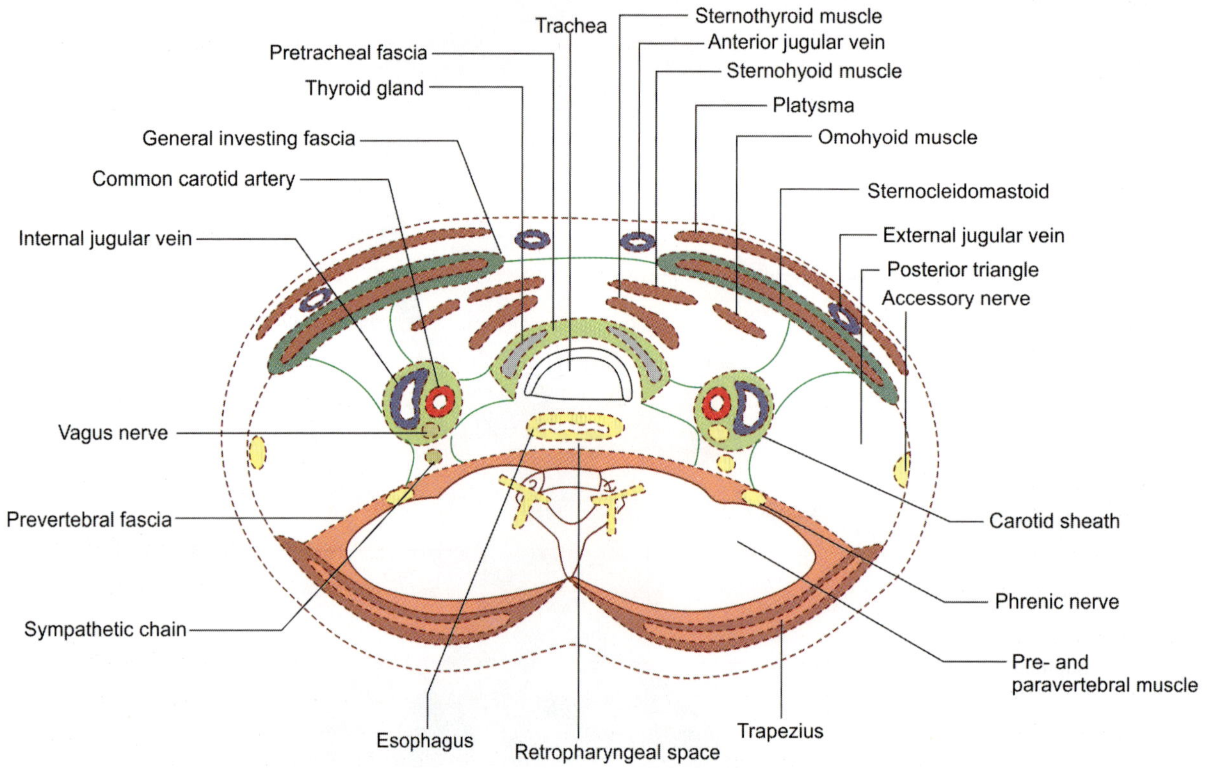

Figure 3.3: Deep cervical fascia—level C_7

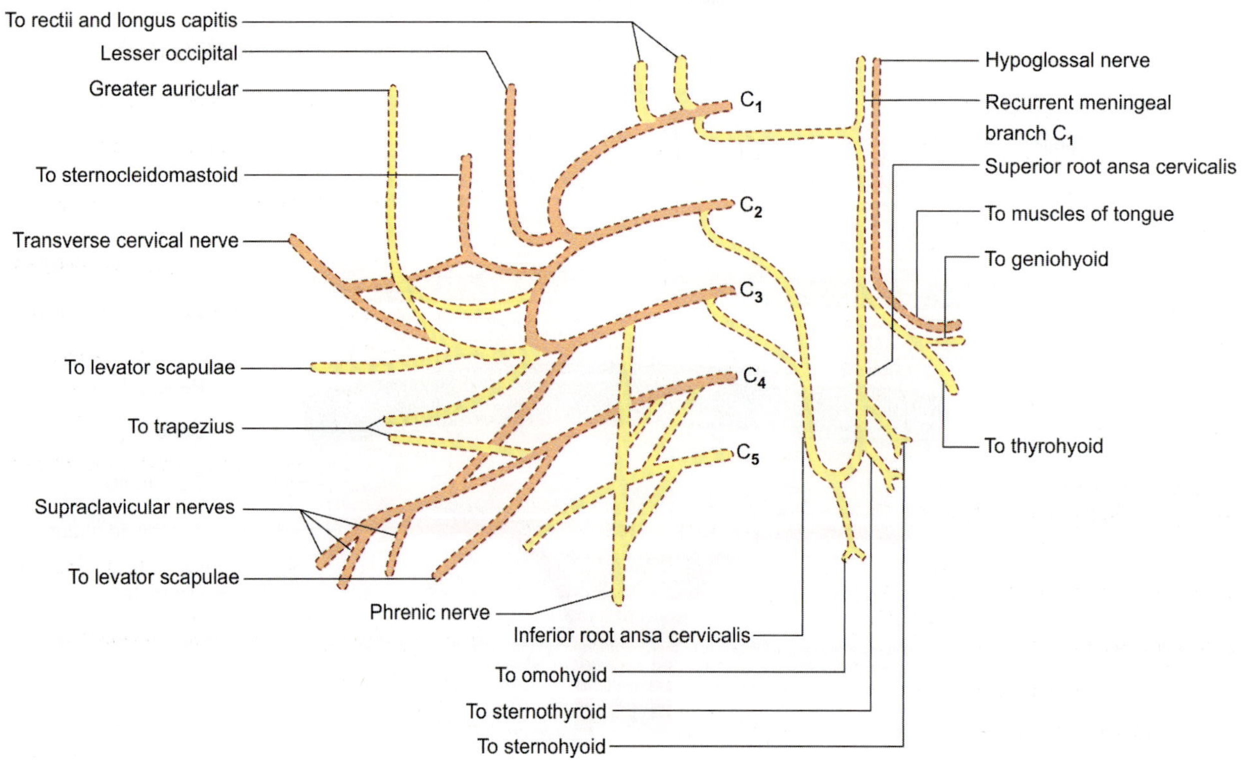

Figure 3.4: Cervical plexus

PLATE 7

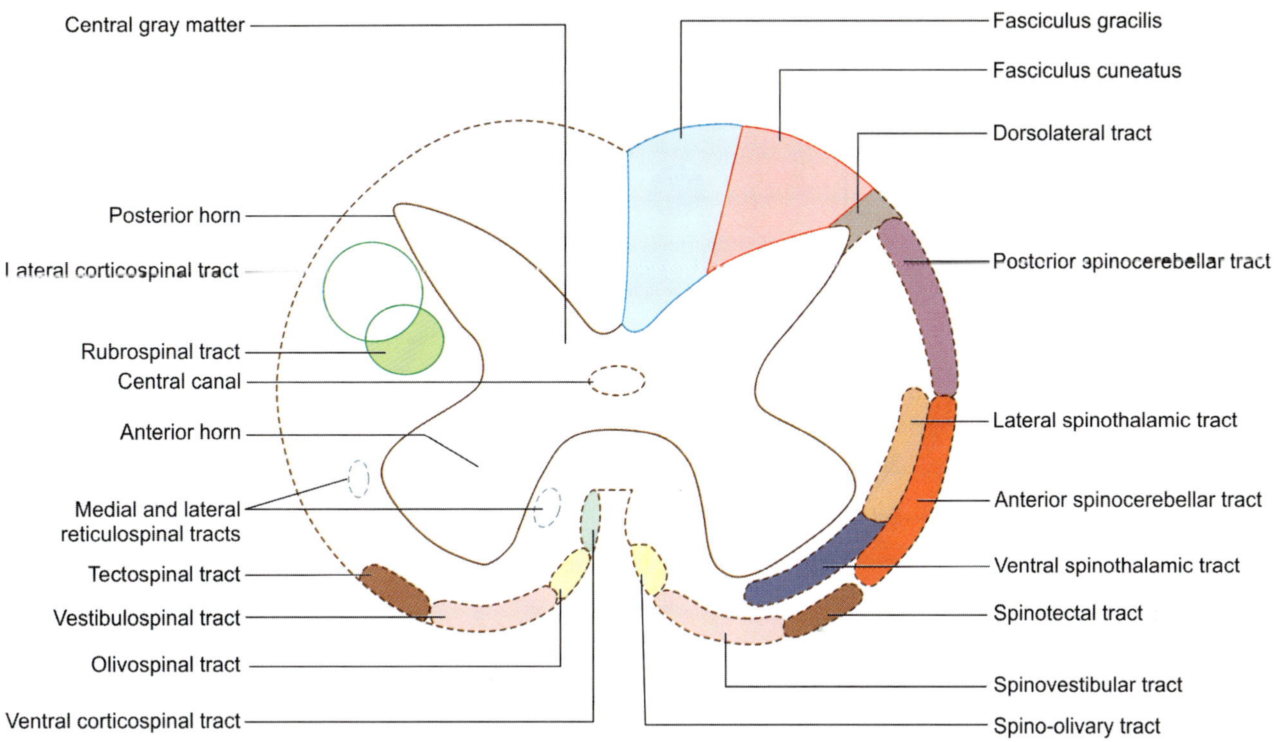

Figure 4.1: Major tracts in spinal cord—descending and ascending

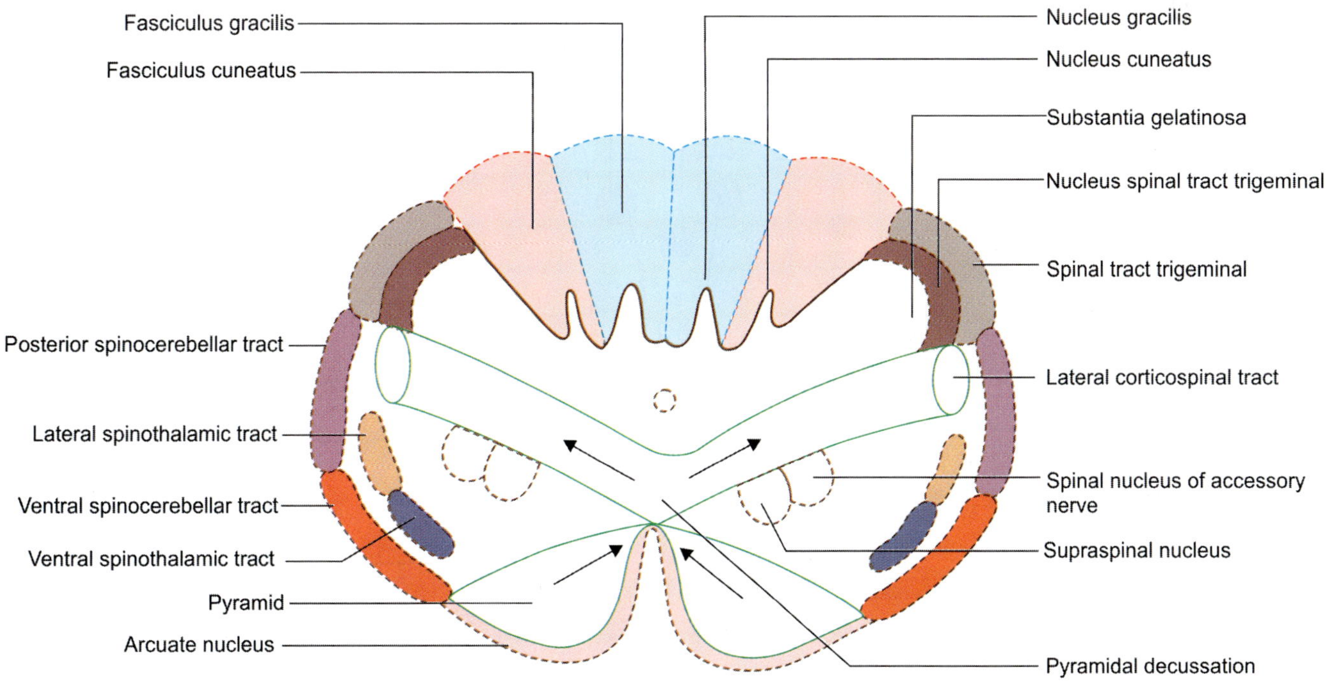

Figure 4.2: Section of medulla—pyramidal decussation

PLATE 8

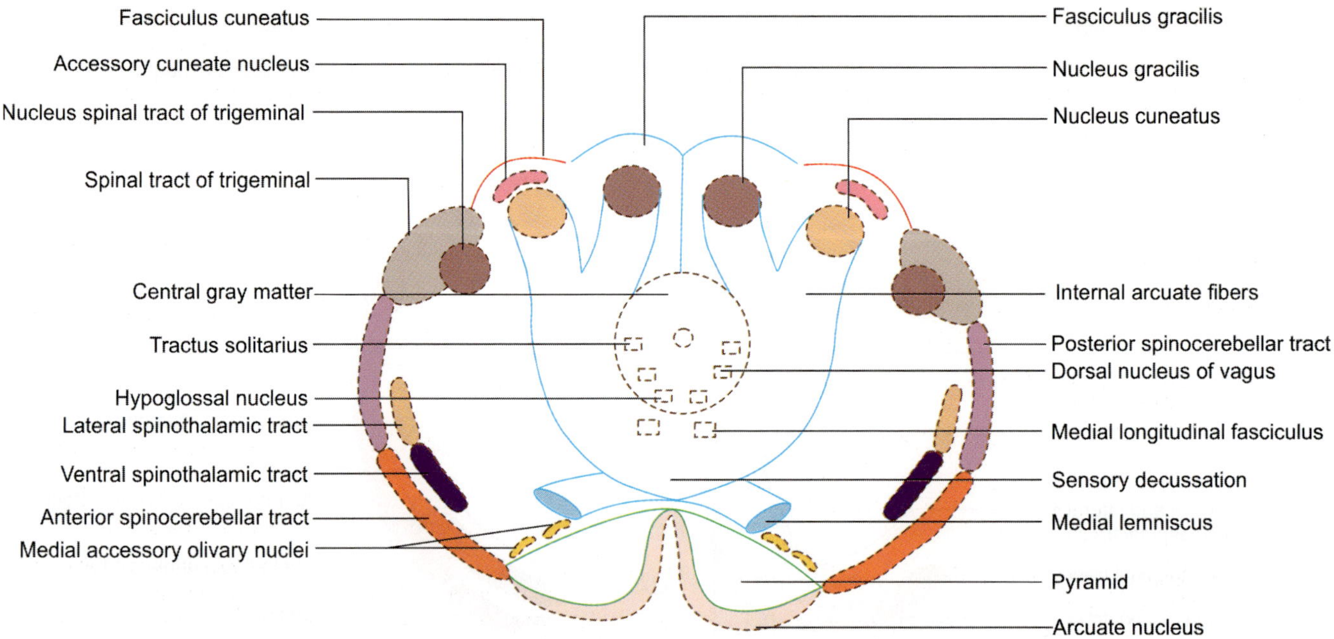

Figure 4.3: Section of medulla—sensory decussation

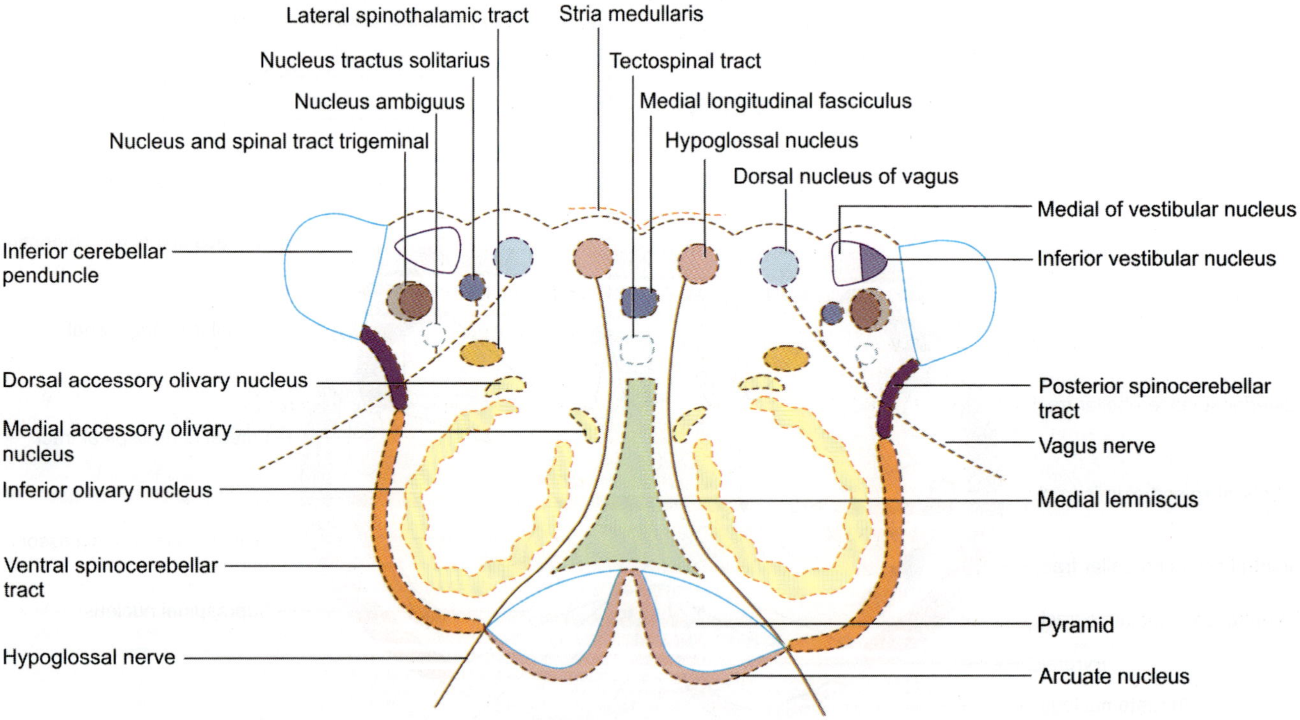

Figure 4.4: Section of medulla—inferior olivary nucleus

PLATE 9

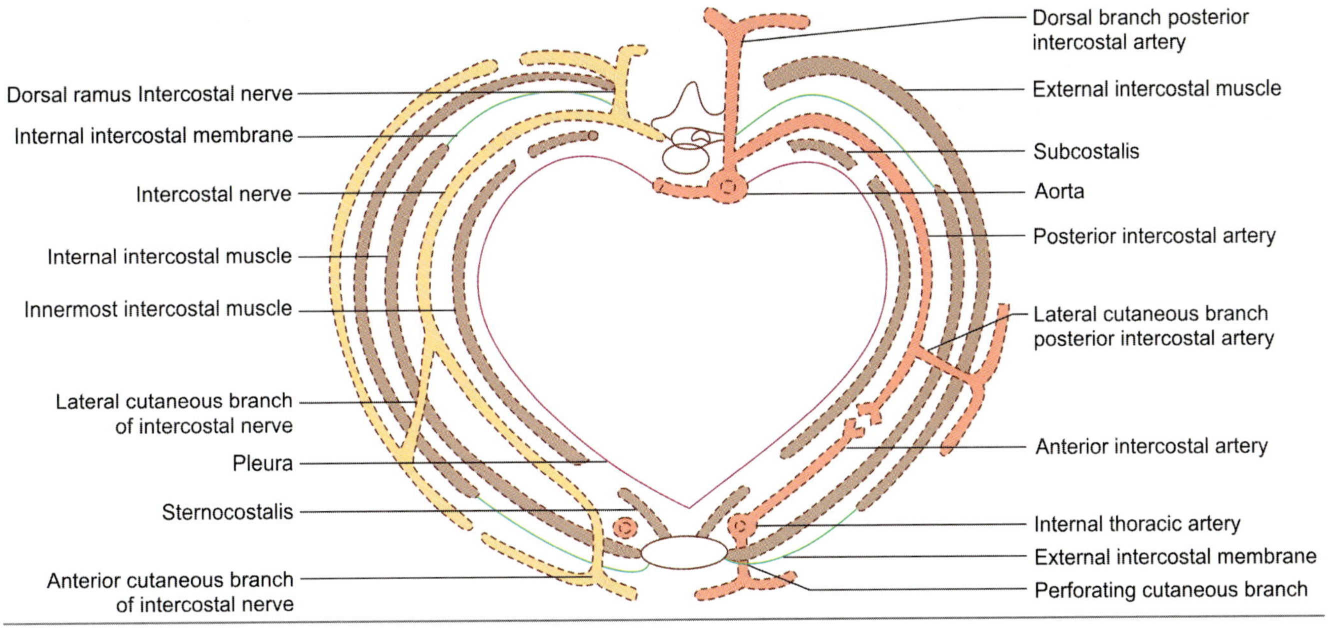

Figure 5.1: Intercostal vessels and nerves

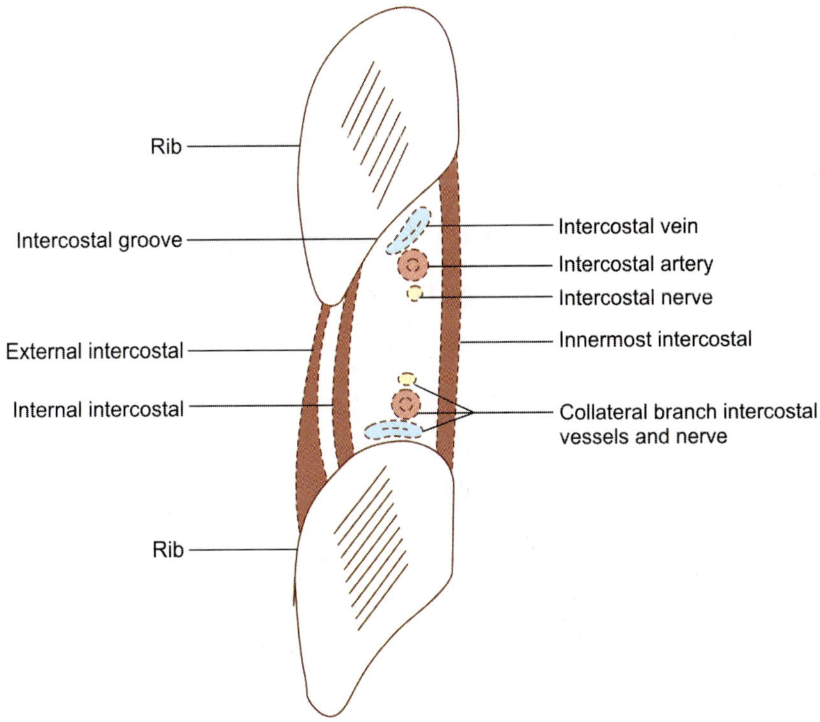

Figure 5.2: Intercostal space—parasagittal section

PLATE 10

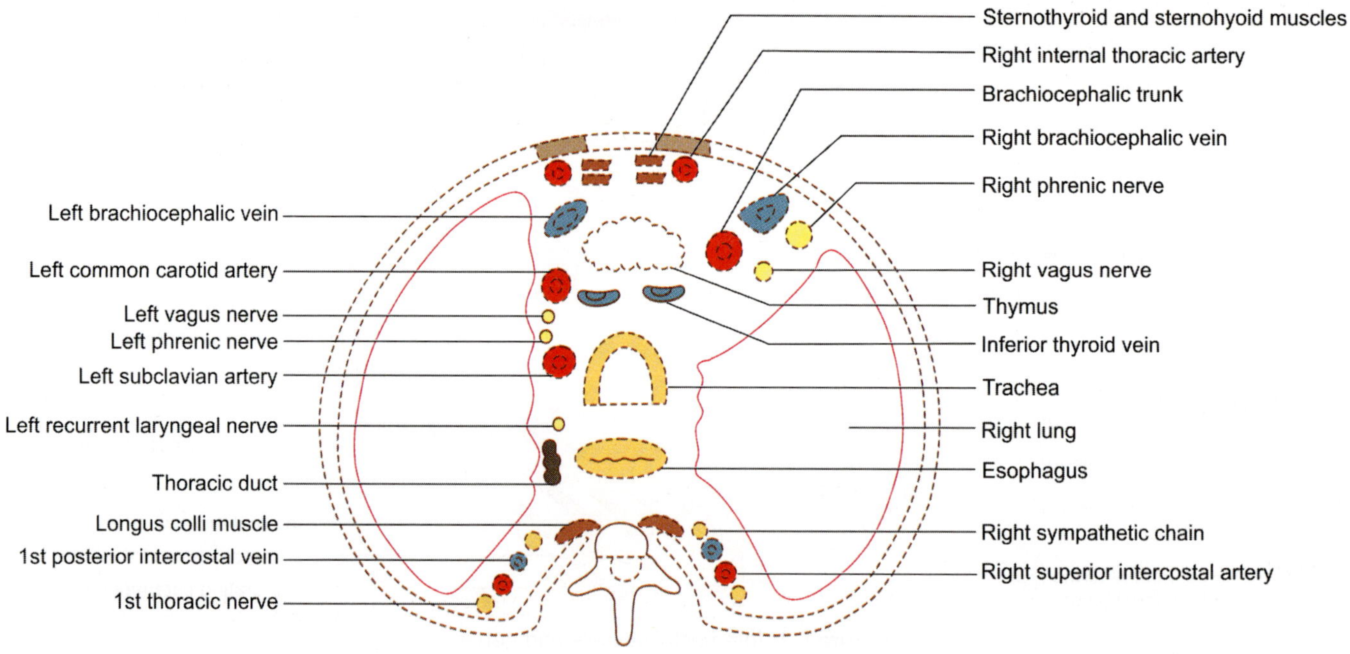

Figure 5.3: Superior mediastinum—TS

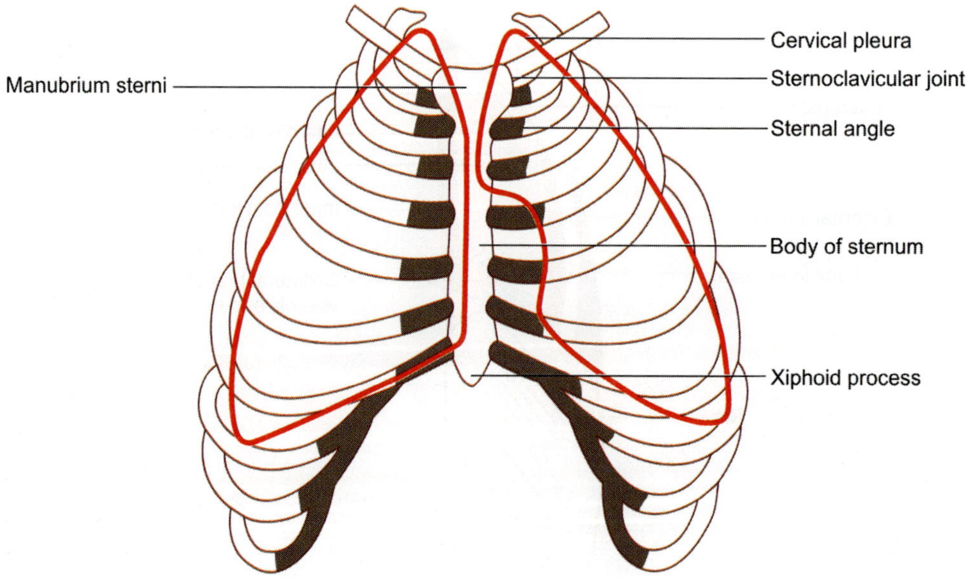

Figure 5.4: Pleural reflections

PLATE 11

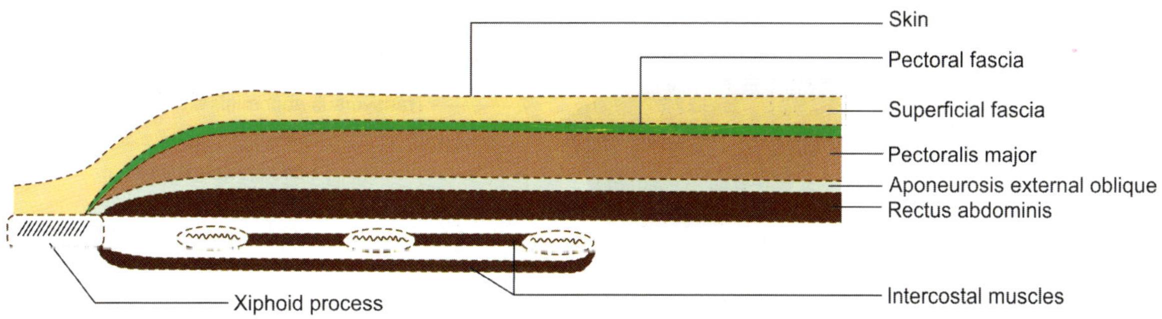

Figure 6.1: Rectus sheath transverse section—above costal margin

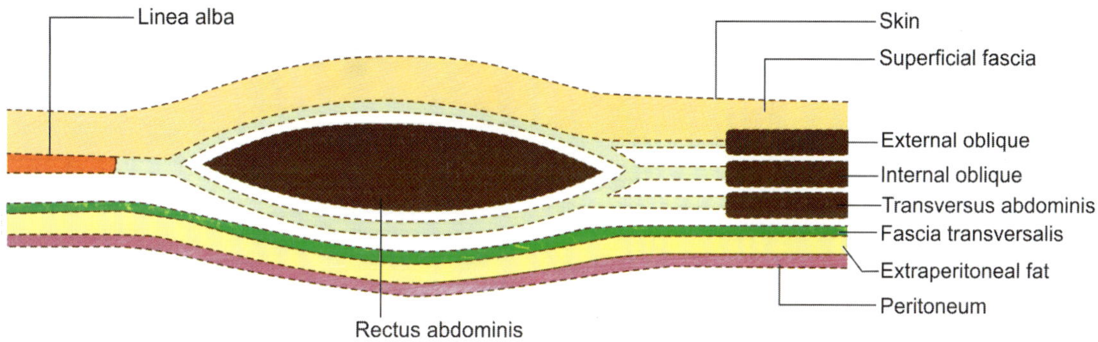

Figure 6.2: Rectus sheath transverse section—between costal margin and anterior superior iliac spine

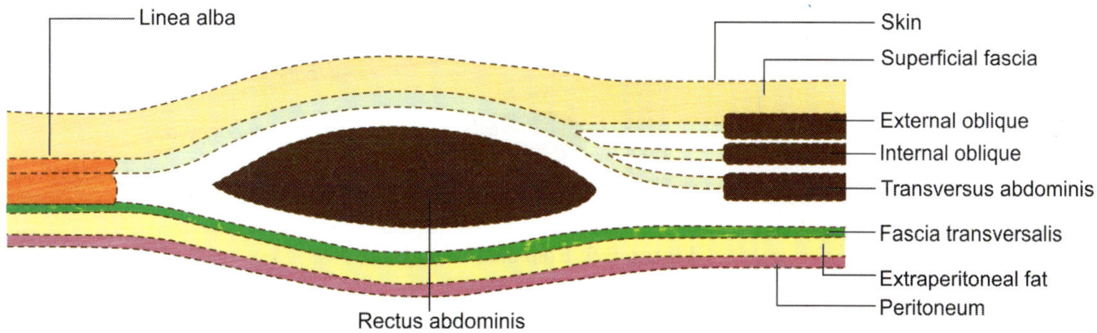

Figure 6.3: Rectus sheath transverse section—between anterior superior iliac spine and pubic symphysis

PLATE 12

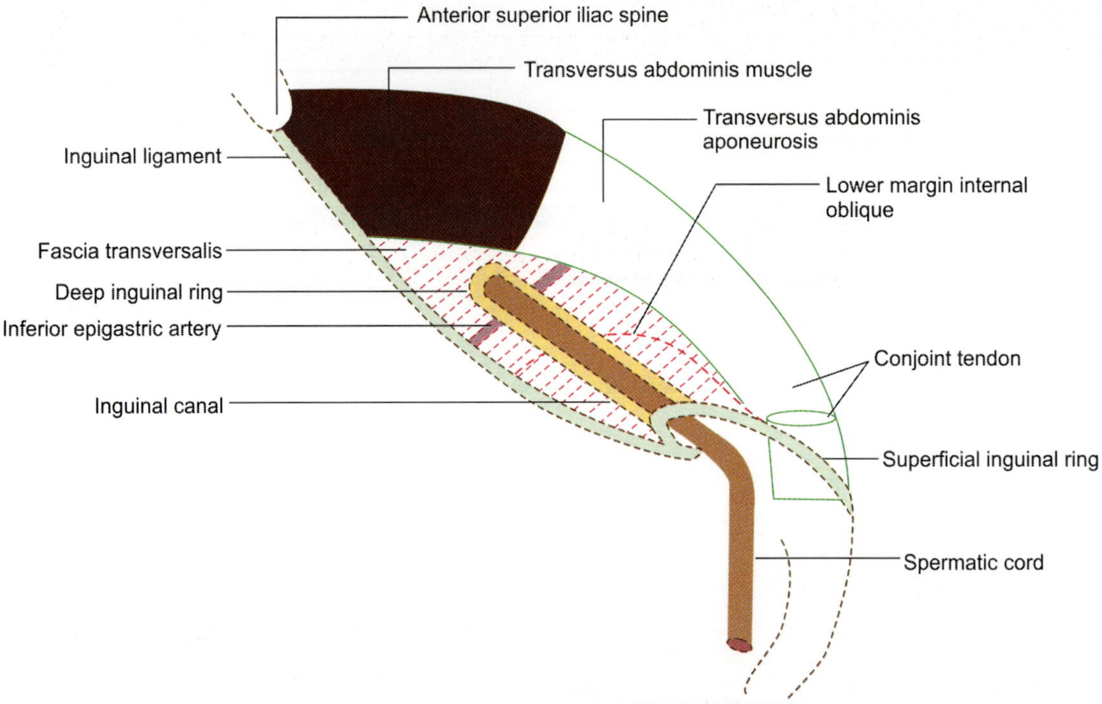

Figure 6.4: Inguinal canal

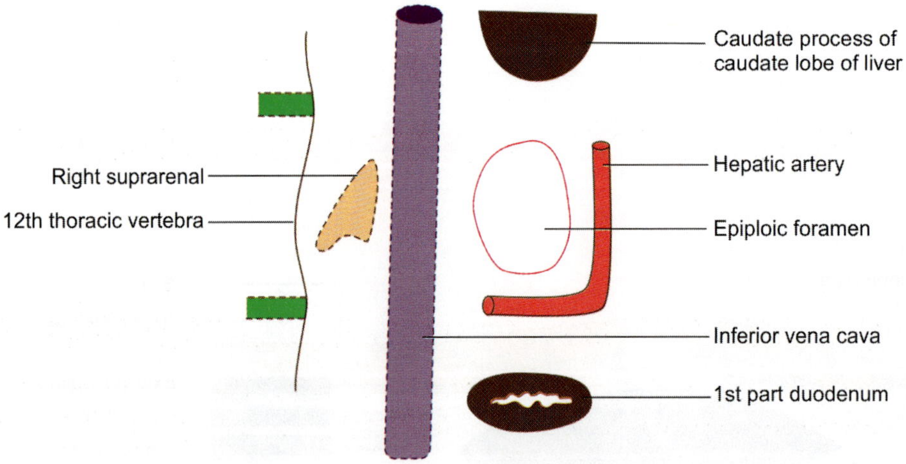

Figure 6.5: Epiploic foramen

CHAPTER 1

Lower Limb

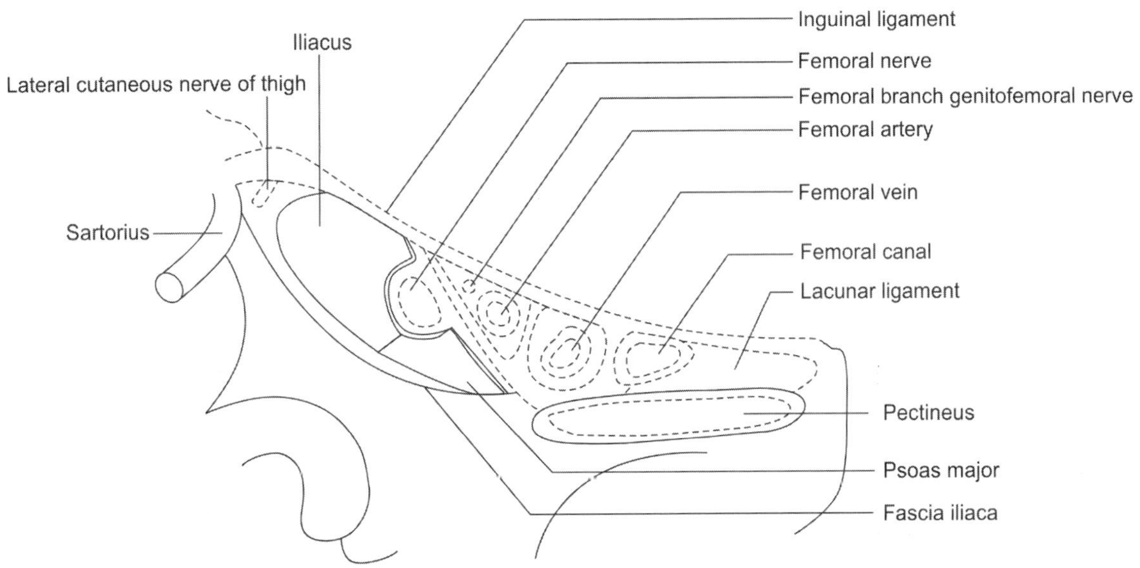

Figure 1.1: Structures passing under inguinal ligament (*For color version, see Plate 1*)

KEY FEATURES

- The space between inguinal ligament and hip bone is divided in two parts:
  - i. Lateral—neuromuscular compartment through which lateral cutaneous nerve of thigh, femoral nerve and iliopsoas muscle passes.
  - ii. Medial—vascular compartment forming femoral sheath between fascia transversalis and fascia iliaca for the passage of femoral vessels.

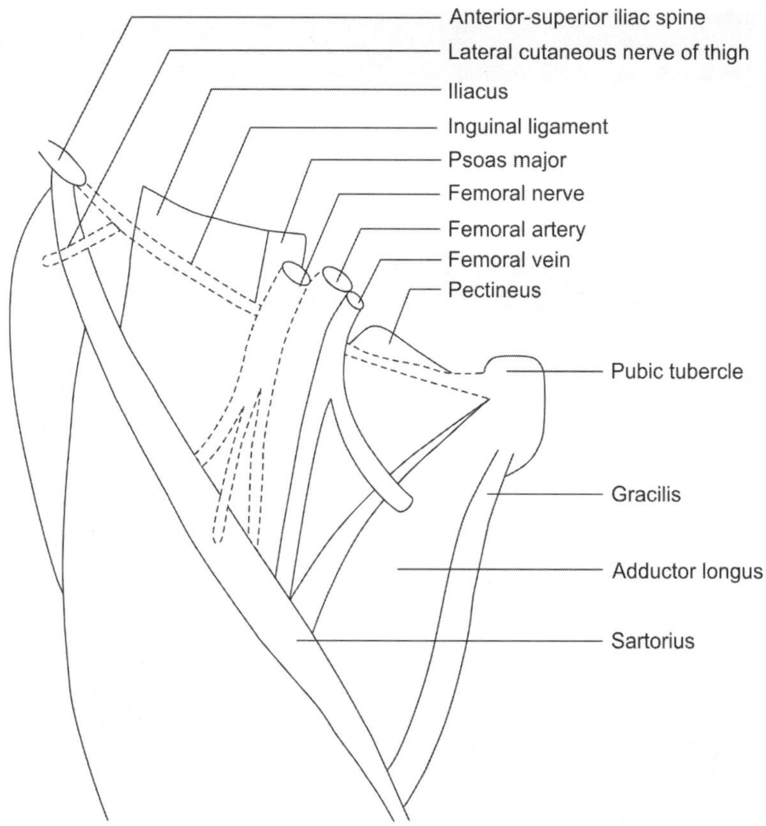

Figure 1.2: Femoral triangle (*For color version, see Plate 1*)

KEY FEATURES

➠ Clinical aspect:

- Femoral pulse can be felt at mid inguinal point just below inguinal ligament.
- Used as a site for intravenous injections.
- Site for catheterization to demonstrate coronary arteries.
- Femoral hernia extends into femoral triangle below and lateral to pubic tubercle.
- Stab injury at the apex of femoral triangle will cut both femoral artery and vein.

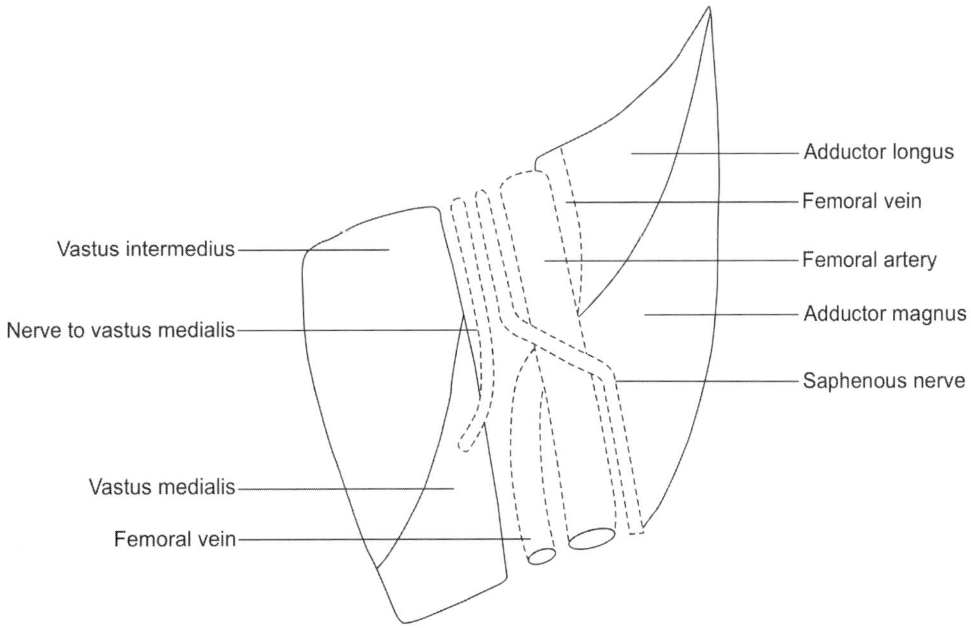

Figure 1.3: Adductor canal (*For color version, see Plate 2*)

KEY FEATURES

- Extends from apex of femoral triangle to the adductor hiatus present in adductor magnus
- Roof faces anteromedially and contains subsartorial plexus of nerves under the sartorius
- Bleeding below knee can be arrested by compressing femoral vessels in adductor canal.

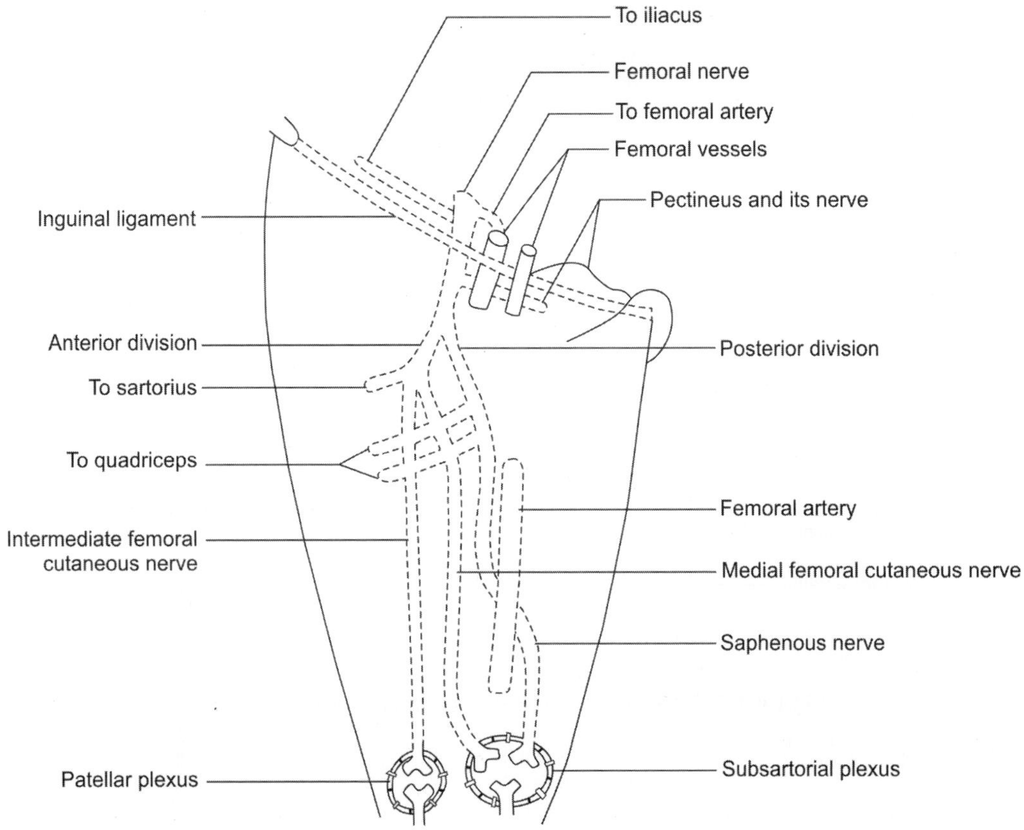

Figure 1.4: Femoral nerve (*For color version, see Plate 2*)

KEY FEATURES

- Root value: Dorsal branches of the ventral rami L2, L3, L4 spinal nerves
- Before entering the femoral triangle gives off branch to iliacus and femoral artery
- Its branching pattern resembles cauda equina
- Participates in the formation of patellar and subsartorial plexus
- The saphenous nerve crosses femoral artery from lateral to medial side in adductor canal
- It supplies both hip and knee joint.

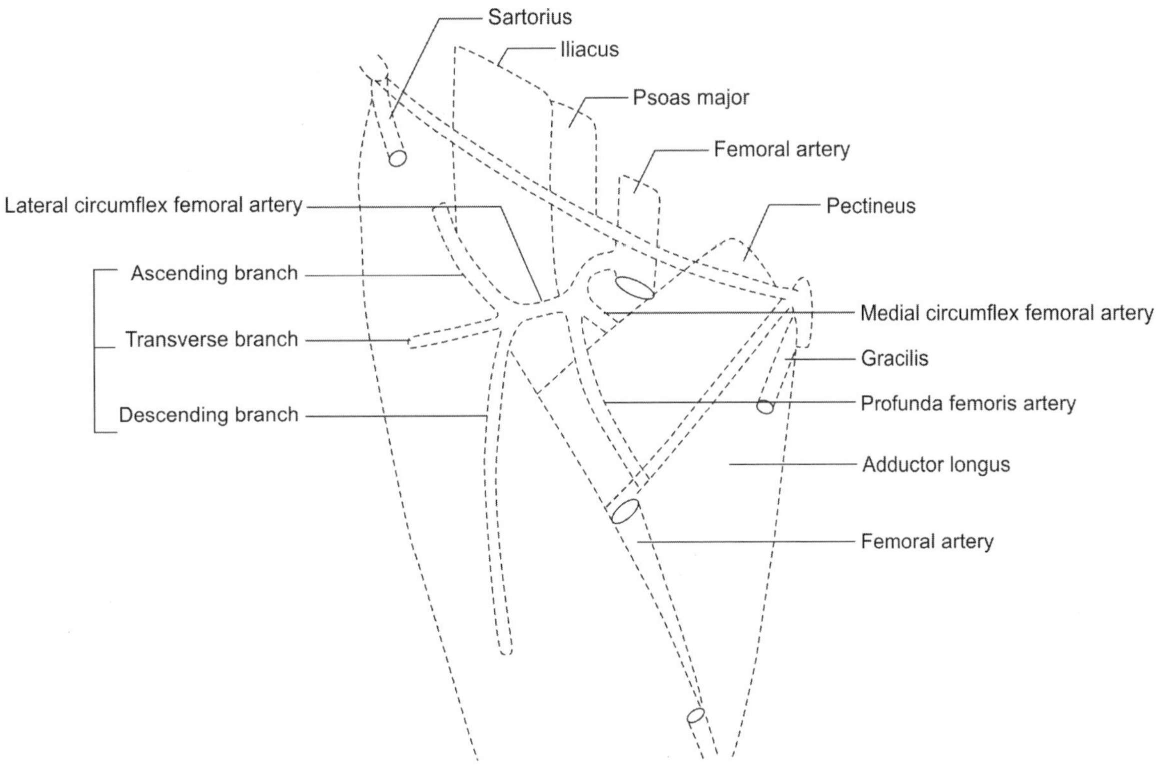

Figure 1.5: Profunda femoris artery—anterior view

KEY FEATURES

- Lateral circumflex femoris artery leaves the femoral triangle under the sartorius muscle
- Medial circumflex femoris artery leaves the femoral triangle between psoas and pectineus muscles
- Profunda femoris artery leaves the femoral triangle between pectineus and adductor longus.

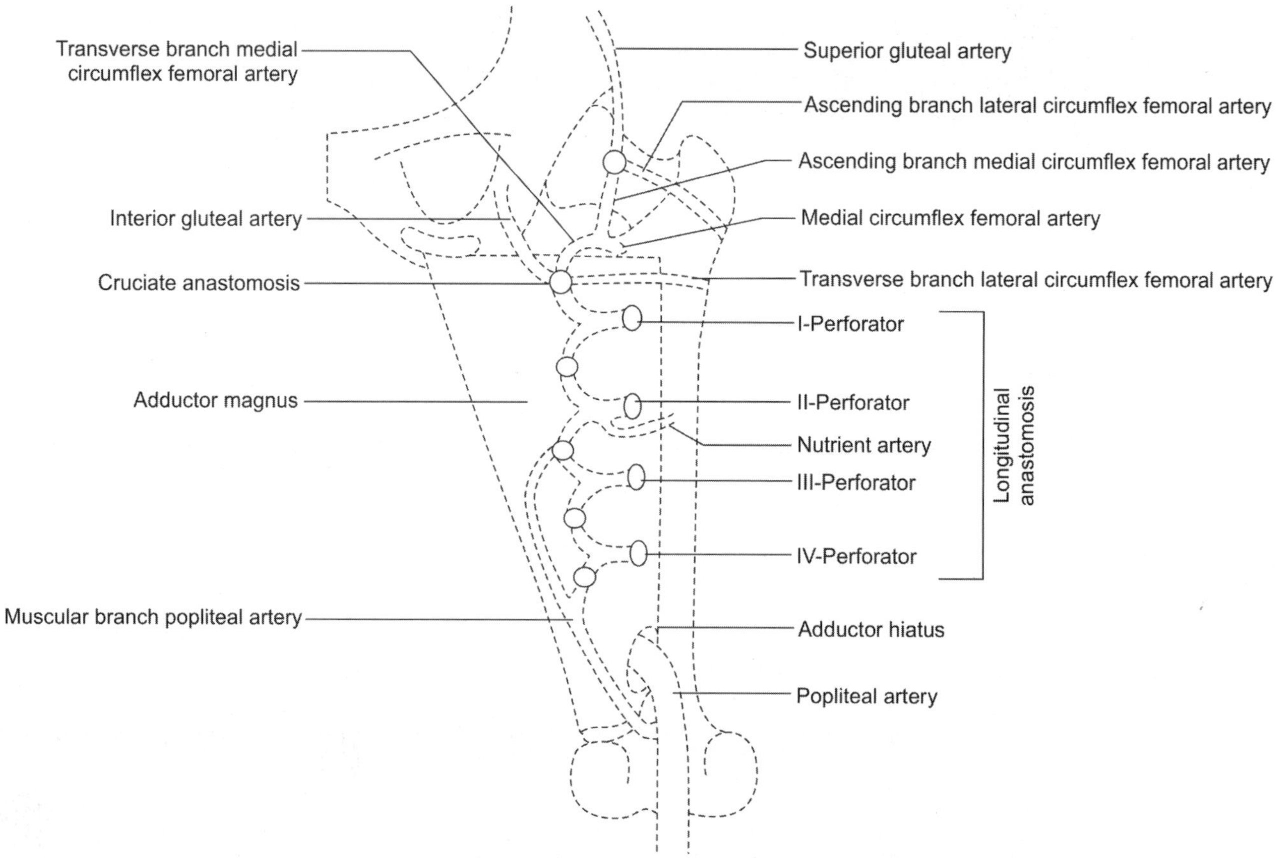

Figure 1.6: Profunda femoris artery—posterior view

KEY FEATURES

- Profunda femoris artery gives three perforating branches and fourth perforator is the continuation of profunda itself in medial compartment of thigh
- These perforators pierce the adductor magnus and enter posterior compartment of thigh
- In association with superior and inferior gluteal arteries form a longitudinal anastomosis.

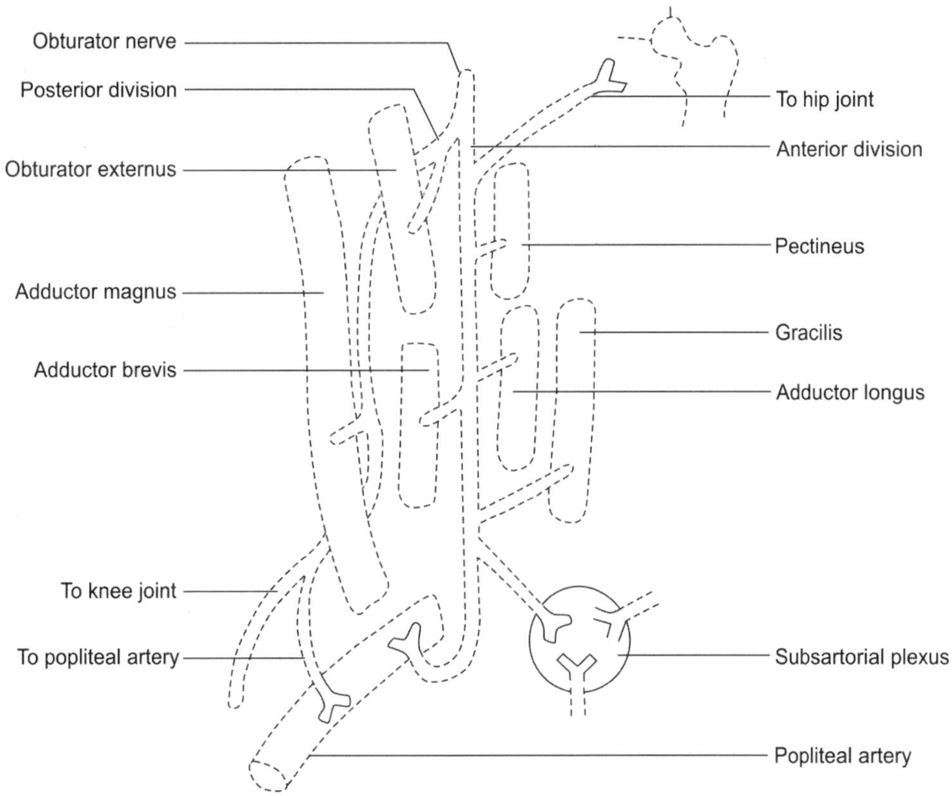

Figure 1.7: Obturator nerve

KEY FEATURES

- Root value: Ventral branches ventral rami L2, L3, L4 spinal nerves
- It is the nerve of adductor muscles
- Enters medial compartment of thigh through obturator canal with obturator artery
- Anterior division supplies knee joint whereas posterior division supplies knee and hip both
- Participates in the formation of subsartorial plexus.

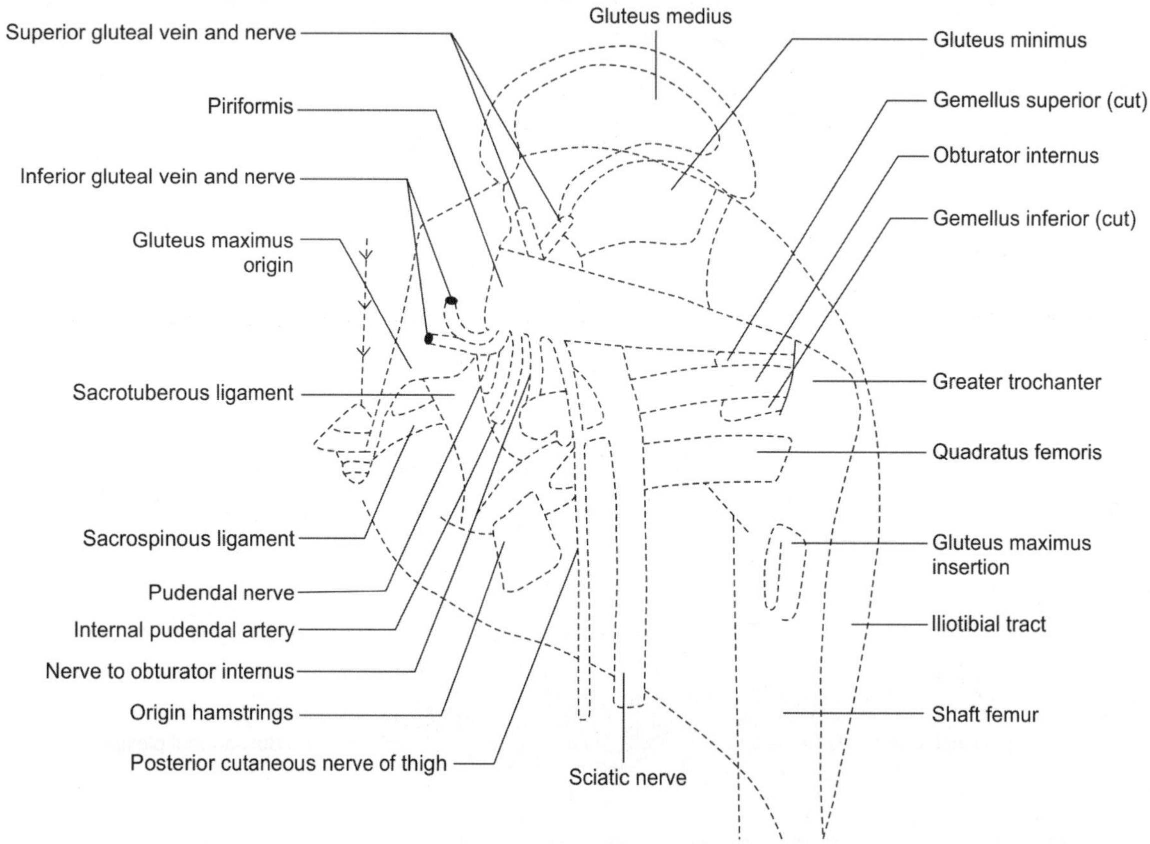

Figure 1.8: Structures under gluteus maximus

KEY FEATURES

- All small muscles of gluteal region are lateral rotators of hip joint
- Intramuscular injections are given in upper lateral quadrant of gluteal region to avoid injury to sciatic nerve
- Sciatic nerve is the thickest nerve of the body and has an artery at the center hence called pregnant nerve
- Pudendal nerve, nerve to obturator internus and internal pudendal artery enter gluteal region through greater sciatic foramen and enter back into pelvis through lesser sciatic foramen
- Gluteus medius is the most powerful abductor of the hip joint.

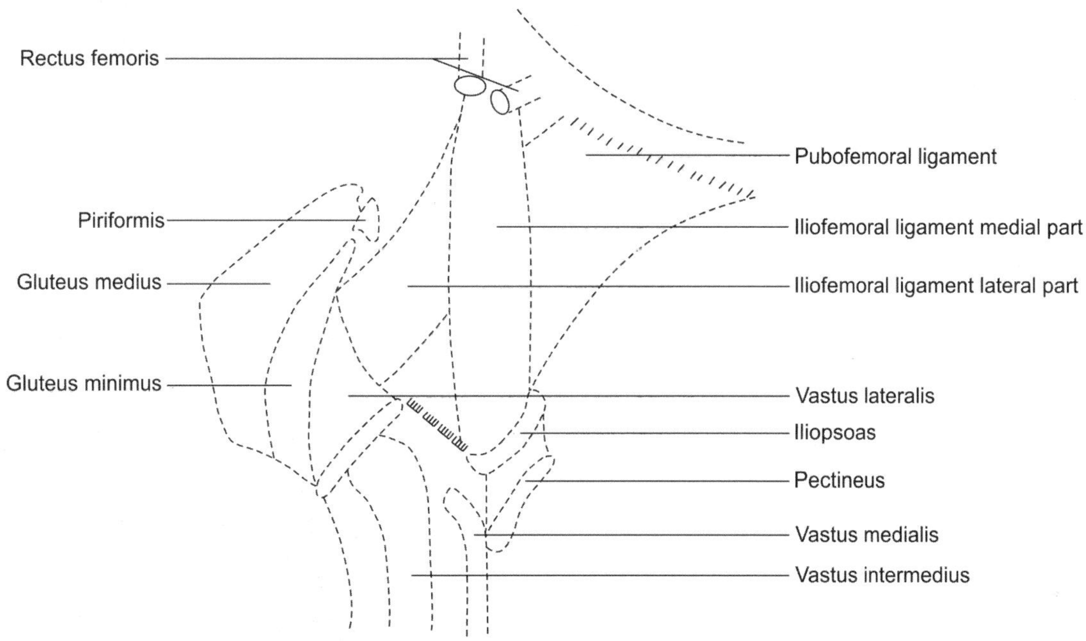

Figure 1.9: Hip joint—anterior view

KEY FEATURES

- Two ligaments reinforce hip joint anteriorly:
  i. Pubofemoral ligament which passes deep into iliofemoral ligament.
  ii. Iliofemoral ligament which extends from anterior inferior iliac spine to inter trochanteric line. It is one of the strongest ligaments of the body and forms the anatomical basis of reduction of posterior dislocation of hip.

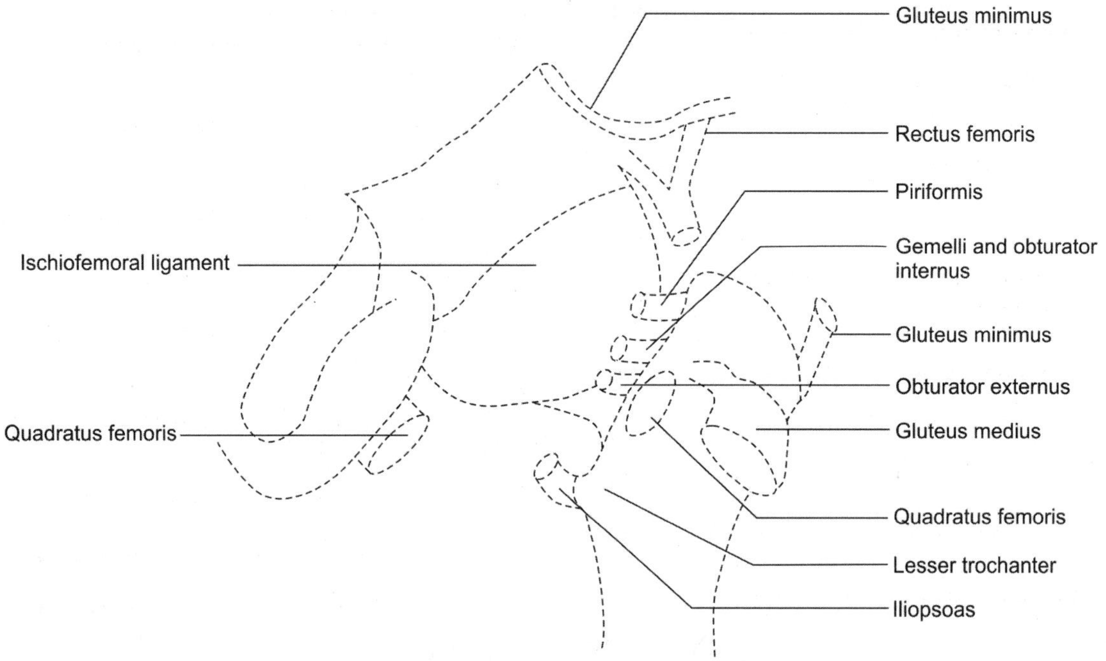

Figure 1.10: Hip joint—posterior view

KEY FEATURES

- One ligament called ischiofemoral which is spiralized
- If there is fracture of neck femur, then the ligament is unspiralized causing lateral rotation of lower limb.

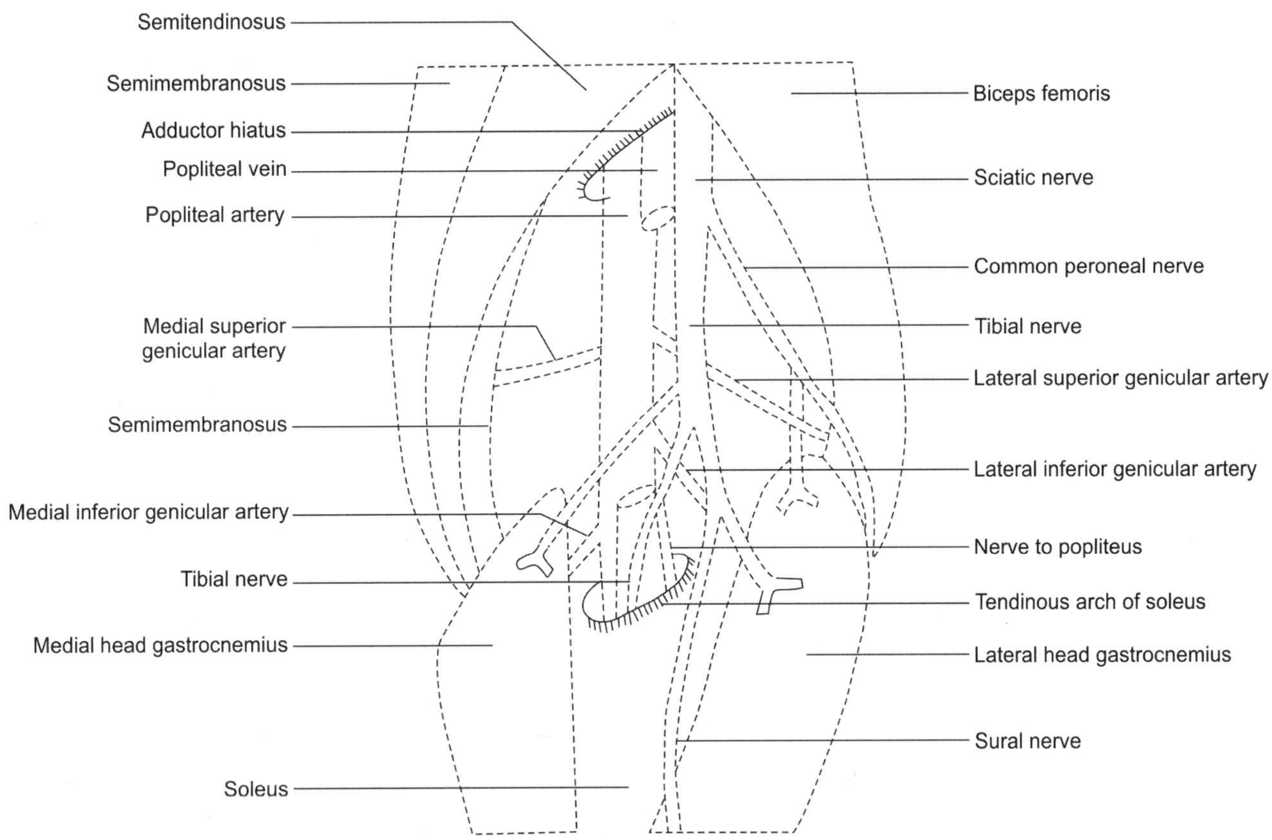

Figure 1.11: Right popliteal fossa

KEY FEATURES

- Located on the posterior aspect of knee
- Bounded above by hamstrings and below by gastrocnemius muscles
- Popliteal artery enters the fossa through adductor hiatus and leaves through soleal arch
- The sciatic nerve divides into tibial and common peroneal branches
- Tibial nerve leaves the fossa along with the artery and common peroneal nerve from lateral side
- The roof is pierced by small saphenous vein and drains into popliteal vein.

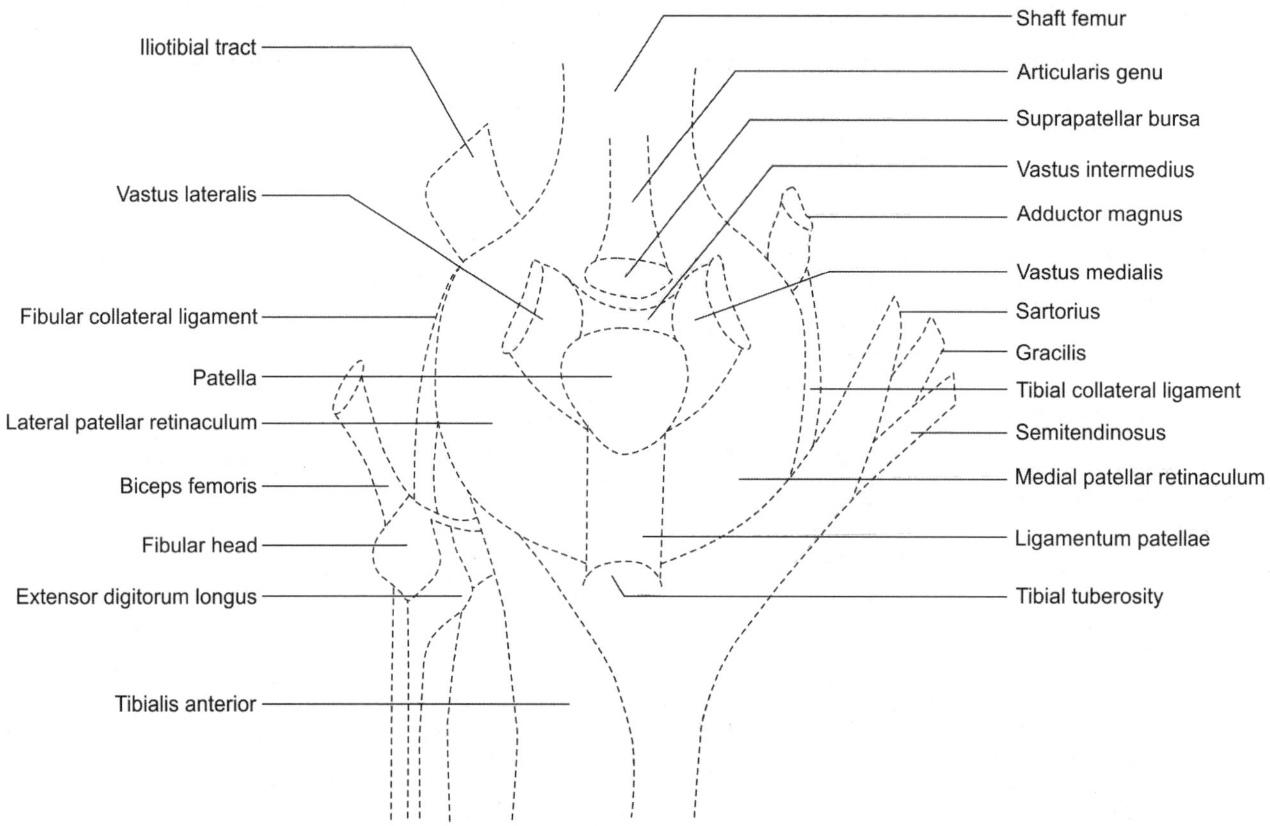

Figure 1.12: Right knee joint—anterior view

KEY FEATURES

- It is a complex variety of condylar synovial joint
- In midline bounded by insertion of quadriceps, patella and ligamentum patella
- On either side by medial and lateral patellar retinaculum
- Above the capsule is deficient and the synovial membrane protrudes as suprapatellar bursa
- This bursa is pulled out during extension by articularis genu, thus preventing injury.

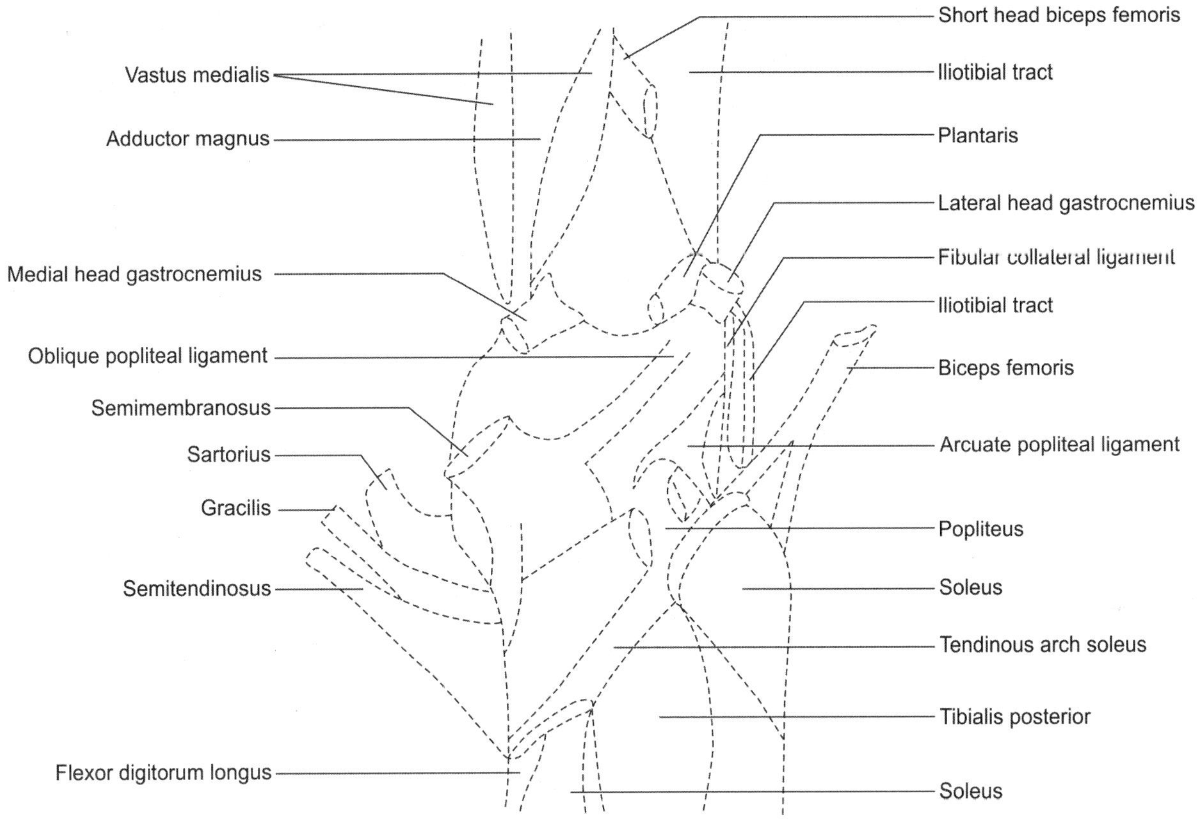

Figure 1.13: Right knee joint—posterior view

KEY FEATURES

- The capsule is reinforced by oblique popliteal ligament which is pierced by middle genicular artery and nerve
- A triangular arcuate popliteal ligament is laterally placed and popliteus muscle passes under it
- The popliteus muscle is intracapsular but extrasynovial and unlocks the knee joint at the beginning of flexion.

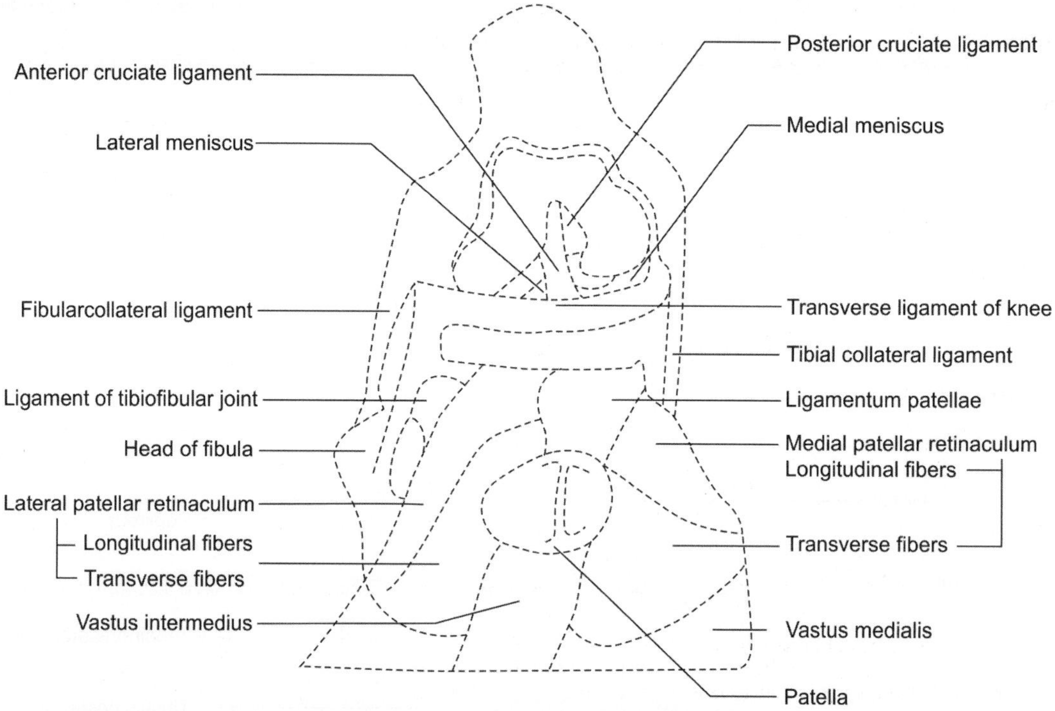

Figure 1.14: Interior right knee joint—anterior view

KEY FEATURES

- Two fibrocartilaginous C-shaped rings called medial and lateral menisci are present
- The medial meniscus is attached to the deep part of tibial collateral ligament medially and to tibia hence fixed and liable to get torn especially in football players
- The lateral meniscus is attached to tibia and to popliteus posteriorly which pulls it during extension thus preventing injury
- The fibular collateral ligament does not fuse with the capsule of knee joint
- The anterior and posterior cruciate ligaments provide anteroposterior stability.

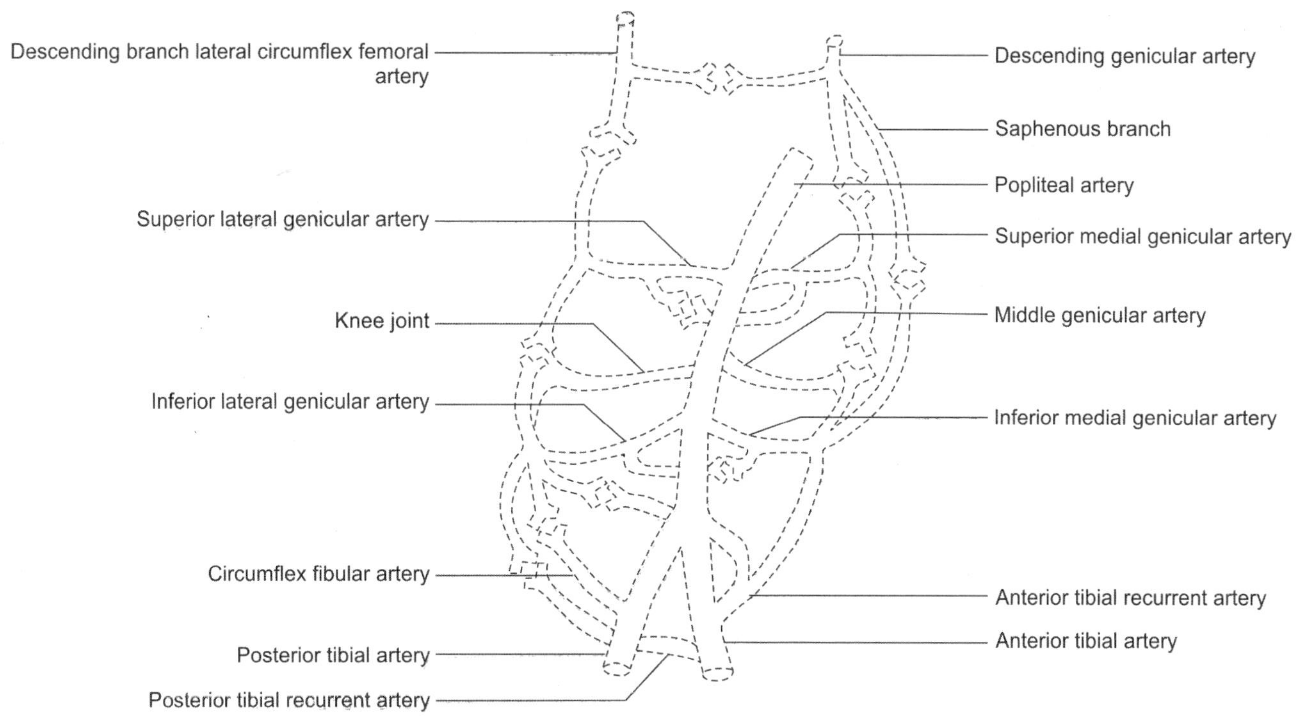

Figure 1.15: Anastomosis around knee joint

KEY FEATURES

- Superior genicular branches of popliteal artery anastomose with genicular branches of femoral artery
- Inferior genicular branches of popliteal artery anastomose with anterior and posterior recurrent tibial arteries and circumflex fibular artery
- This anastomosis is essential for maintaining circulation in leg and foot during flexion of knee.

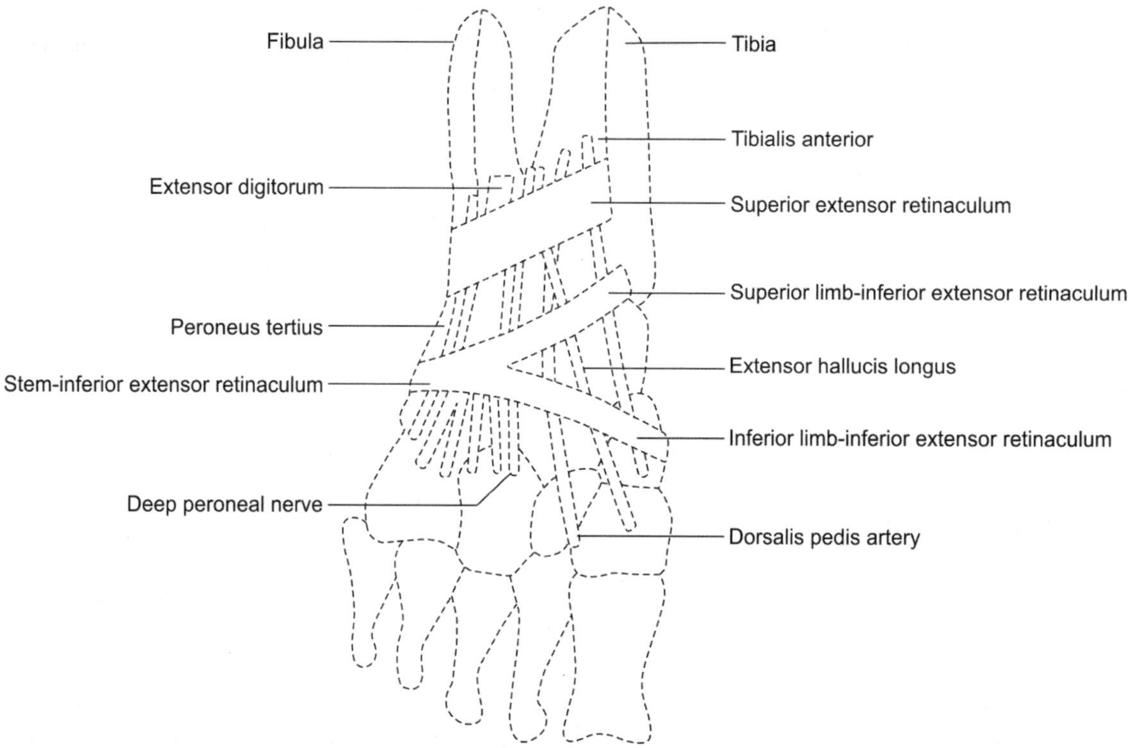

Figure 1.16: Extensor retinaculum

KEY FEATURES

- It is modified deep fascia and act as retention bands to keep the tendons, vessels and nerves in position
- Superior extensor retinaculum is a single band whereas inferior is a Y- shaped band open medially
- If both the retinaculum is cut vertically the tendon/s jumps out on dorsiflexion leading to bow stringing of the tendon.

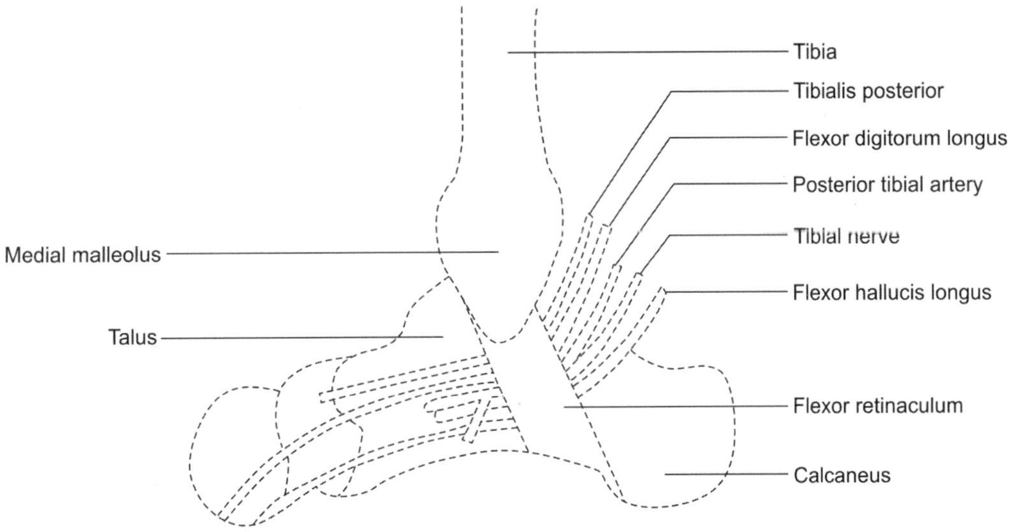

Figure 1.17: Flexor retinaculum

KEY FEATURES

- It forms an osteo-fascial tunnel for the passage of tendons, vessels and nerves from posterior compartment of leg to sole of the foot
- It changes the direction of pull of the muscles.

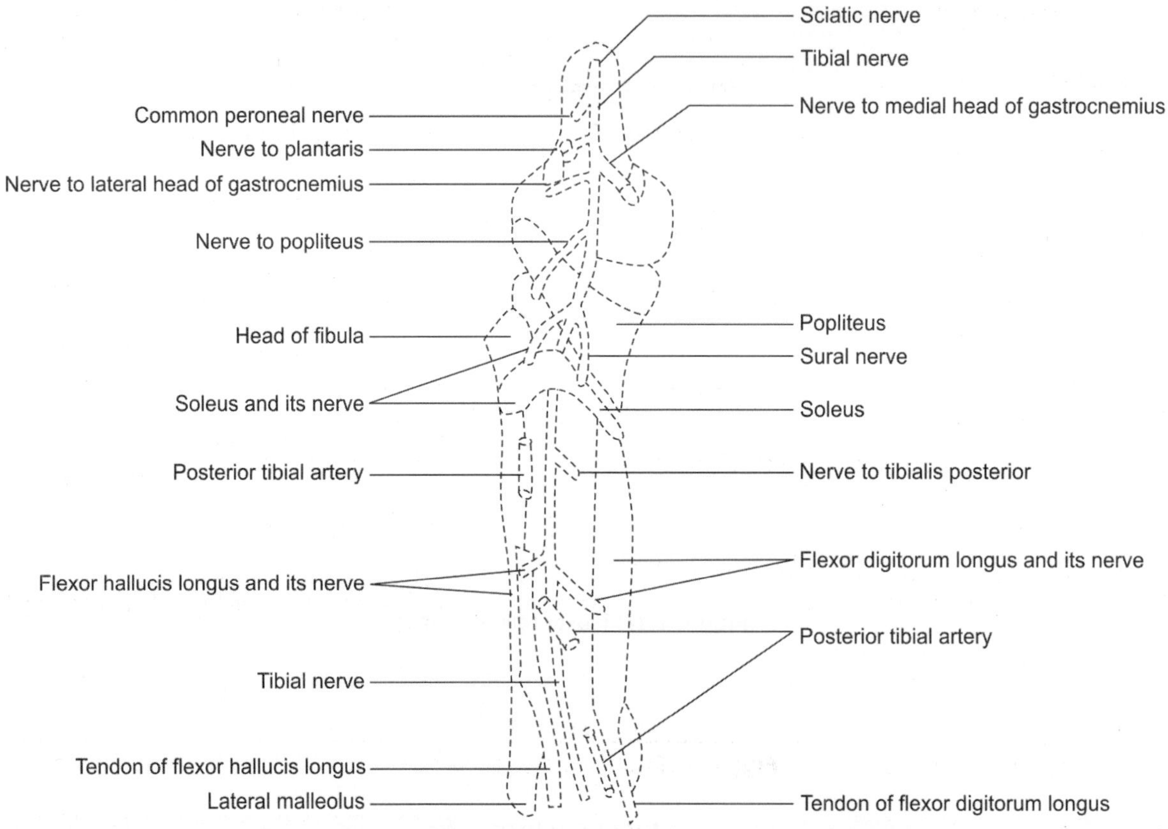

Figure 1.18: Tibial nerve

KEY FEATURES

- Terminal branch of sciatic nerve which enters the posterior compartment of leg under the soleal arch
- It supplies the plantar flexors and enters sole under the cover of flexor retinaculum
- If injured will cause pes calcaneous due to unopposed action of dorsiflexors.

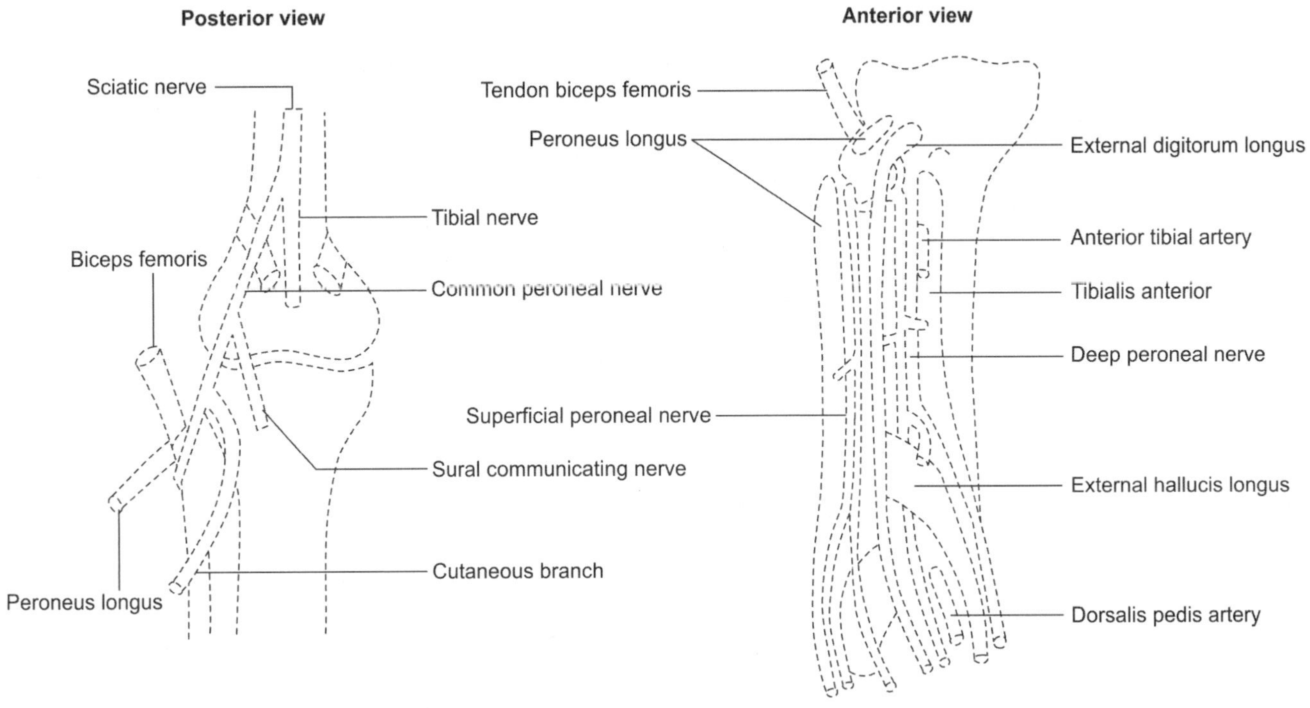

Figure 1.19: Common peroneal nerve

KEY FEATURES

- Terminal branch of sciatic nerve
- Enters lateral compartment by winding around the neck of fibula
- Divides into superficial and deep peroneal nerves
- Superficial branch supplies peroneal group of muscles (evertors of foot)
- Deep branch enters anterior compartment and supplies dorsiflexors of foot
- Injury to common peroneal nerve at neck of fibula causes foot drop and loss of eversion.

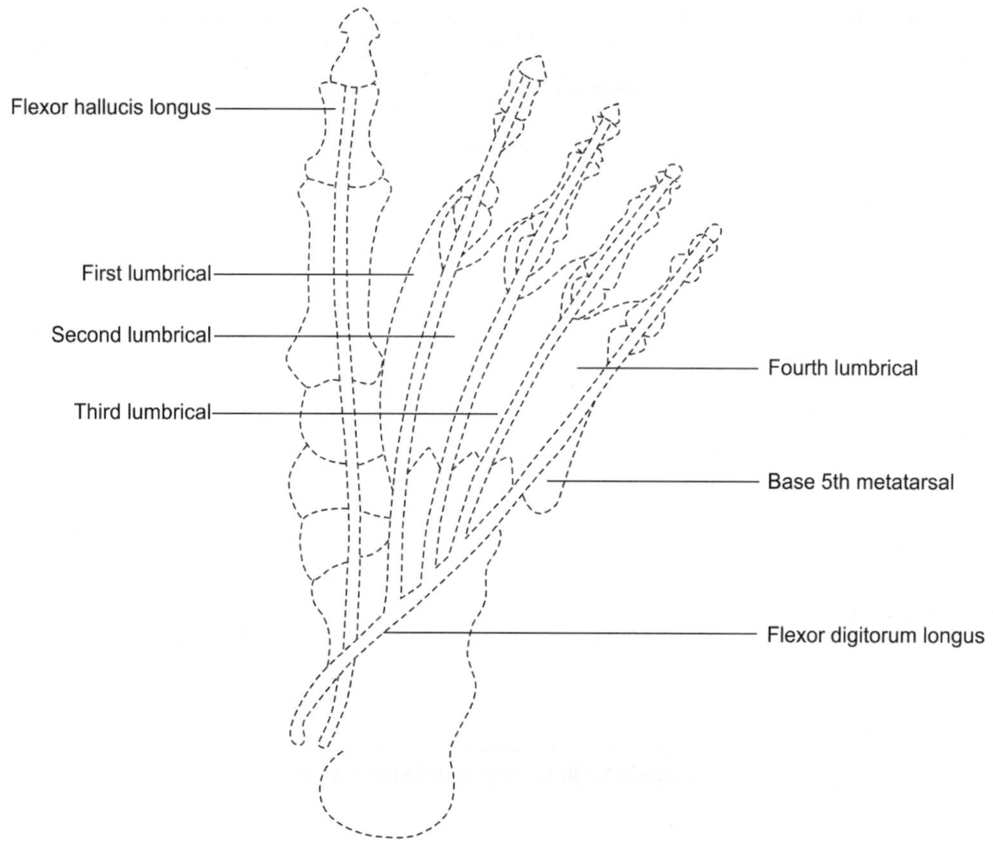

Figure 1.20: Lumbricals

KEY FEATURES

- Arise from the tendons of flexor digitorum longus
- First lumbrical is unipennate and the rest are bipennate
- Get inserted into dorsal digital expansion along with interossei
- First lumbrical is supplied by medial plantar nerve and rest by deep branch of lateral plantar nerve
- Action: Plantar flexion at the metatarsophalangeal joints and extension at interphalangeal joints.

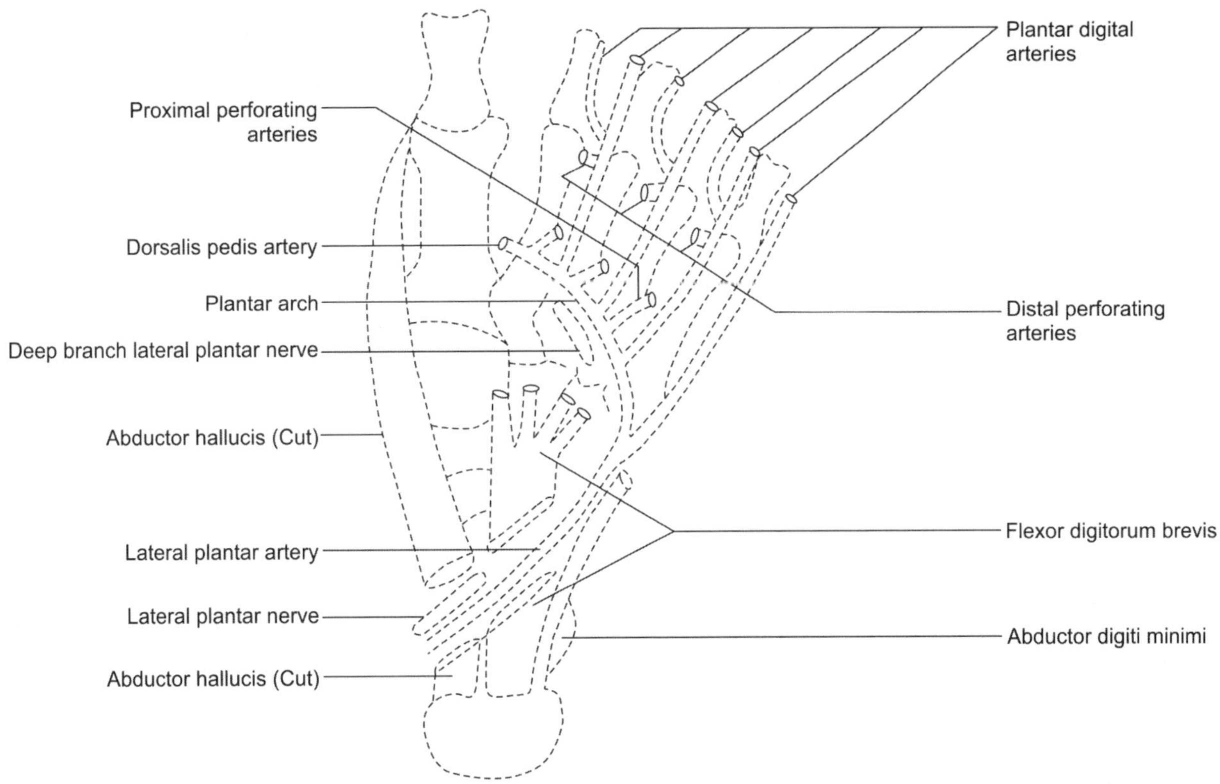

Figure 1.21: Plantar arch—arterial

KEY FEATURES

- Lateral plantar artery is one of the terminal branches of posterior tibial artery
- Enters sole from medial side, runs laterally to reach the base of 5th metatarsal
- Then curves medially to reach 1st interosseous space to anastamose with dorsalis pedis artery to complete the plantar arch
- It gives off three proximal perforating arteries and four plantar digital arteries.

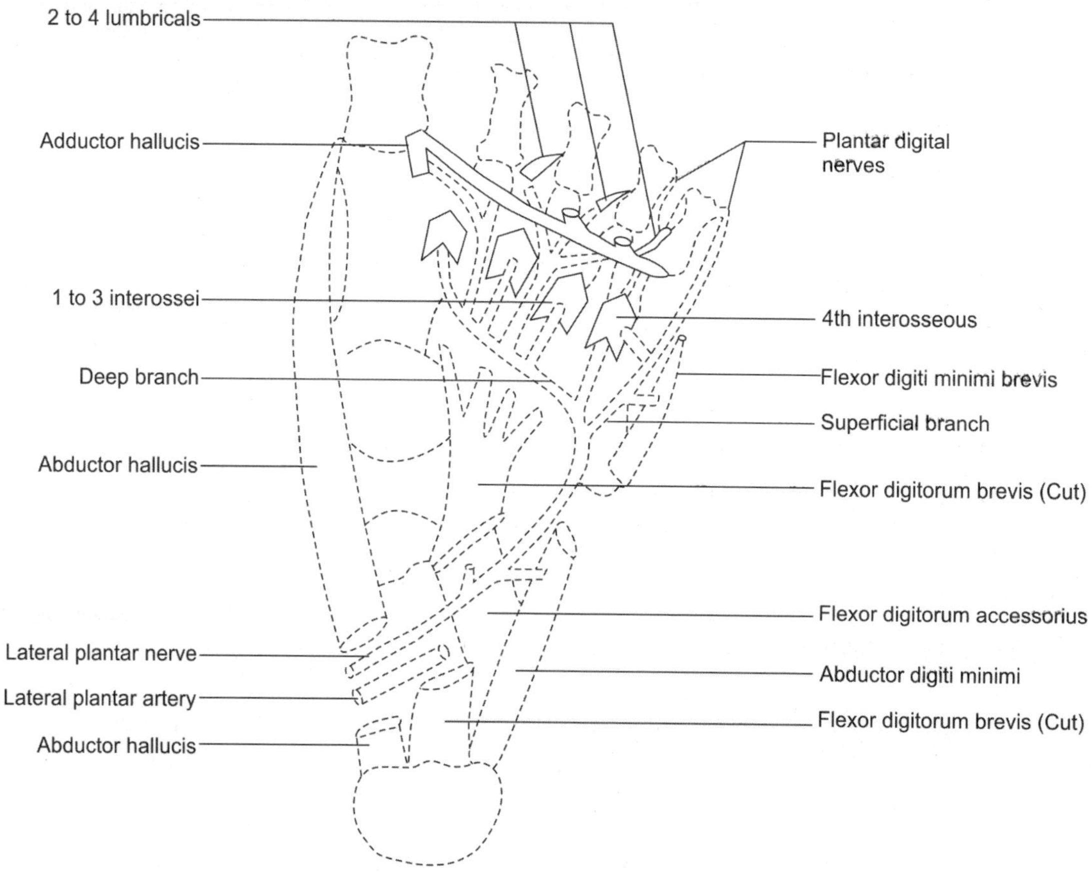

Figure 1.22: Lateral plantar nerve

KEY FEATURES

- Accompanies lateral plantar artery which is lateral to the nerve
- Runs laterally to reach 5th metatarsal base
- Then, turns medially along with lateral plantar artery
- Ends by supplying 1st plantar interosseous muscle
- It supplies all small muscles of foot except abductor hallucis and flexor digitorum brevis.

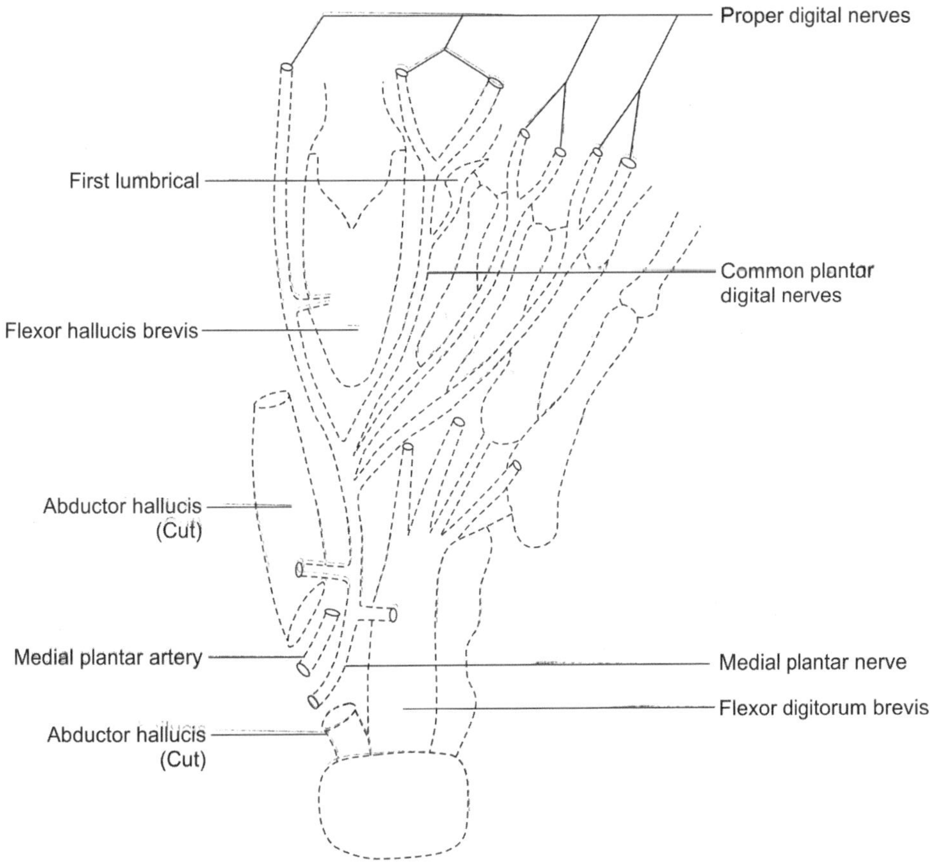

Figure 1.23: Medial plantar nerve

KEY FEATURES

- Enters sole of foot from medial side accompanied by medial plantar artery
- It runs forward and ends by supplying digits
- It only supplies abductor hallucis and flexor digitorum brevis.

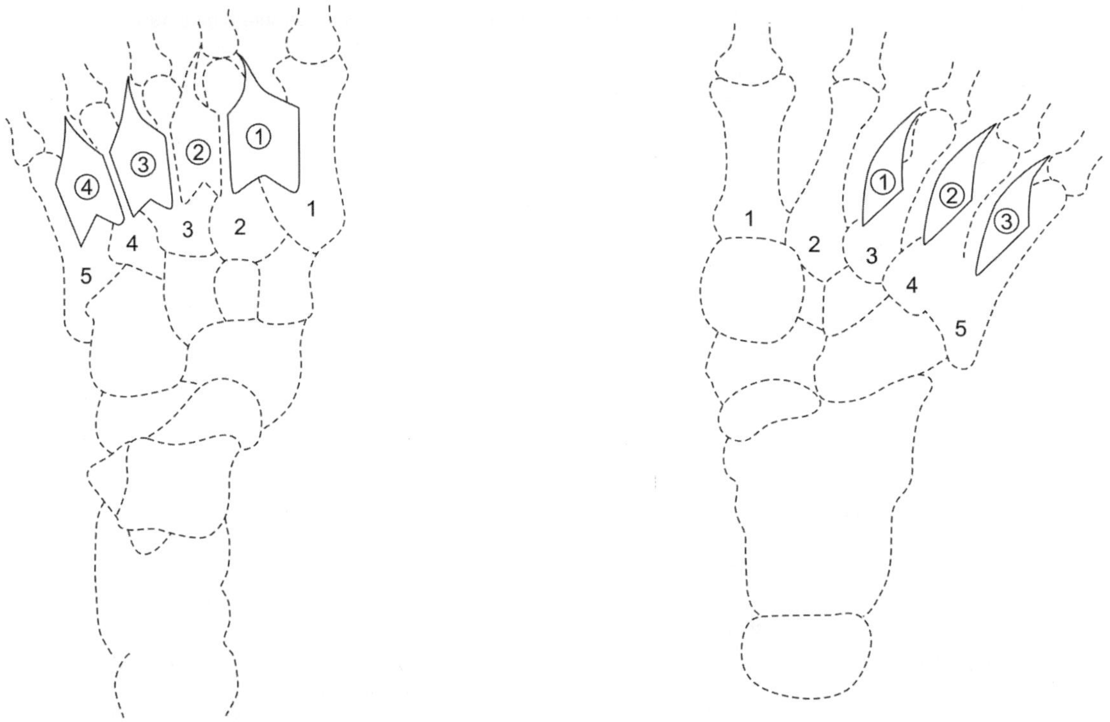

Figure 1.24: Interossei—dorsal and plantar

KEY FEATURES

- Plantar interossei—three in number and bipennate and are adductors of toes
- Dorsal interossei—four in number and unipennate and are abductors of toes
- All interossei are supplied by deep branch lateral plantar nerve except 4th dorsal and 3rd plantar interossei which are supplied by superficial branch lateral plantar nerve.

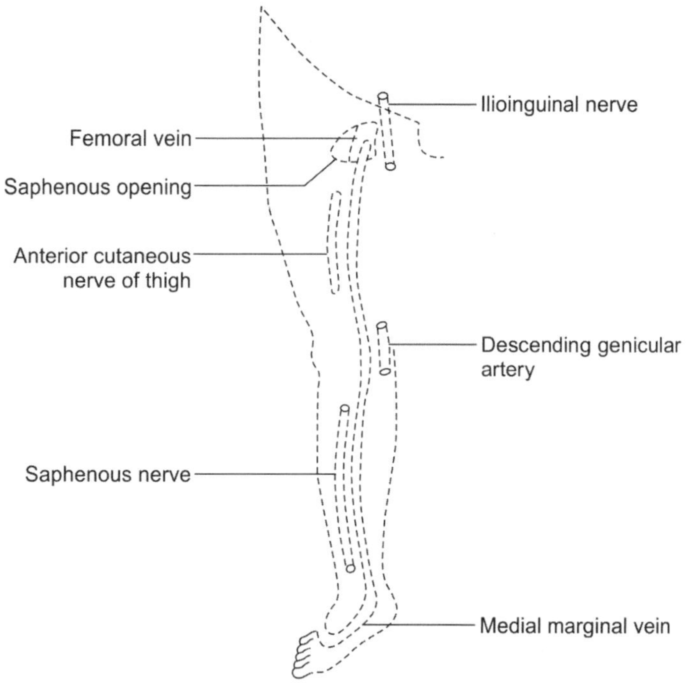

Figure 1.25: Great saphenous vein

KEY FEATURES

- Longest vein of the body
- Begins as the continuation of the medial end of the dorsal venous arch
- Near termination it pierces cribriform fascia, passes through saphenous opening and drains into femoral vein
- It is accompanied by saphenous nerve in leg, descending genicular artery at knee, anterior cutaneous nerve of thigh in front of thigh and ilioinguinal nerve near termination
- It communicates with deep veins through perforators and both have valves
- Due to the defect in the valves the great saphenous vein becomes tortuous leading to varicosity.

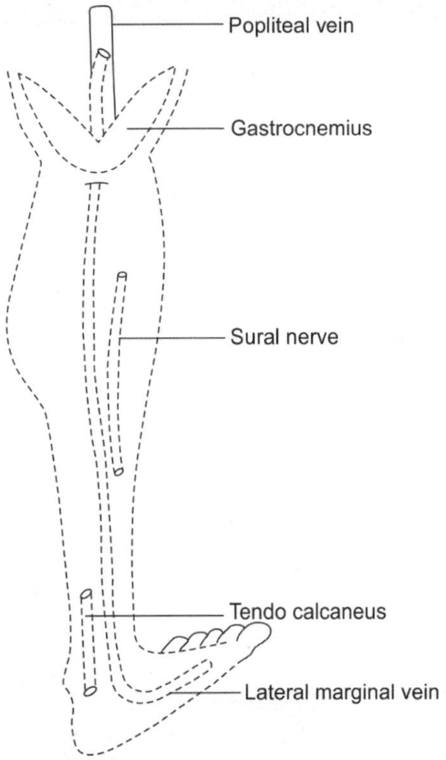

Figure 1.26: Small saphenous vein

KEY FEATURES

- Begins as the continuation of the lateral end of the dorsal venous arch
- Near termination it pierces roof of the popliteal fossa and drains into popliteal vein
- It ascends along the lateral margin of tendo calcaneus and is accompanied by sural nerve.

CHAPTER 2

Upper Limb

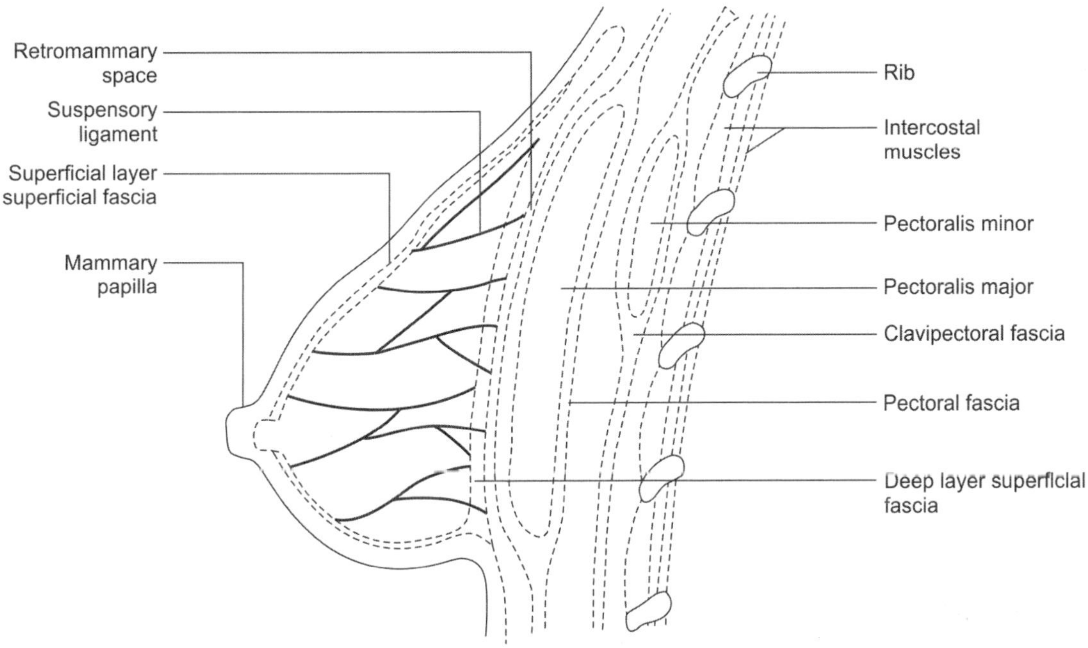

Figure 2.1: Mammary gland—relations (*For color version, see Plate 3*)

KEY FEATURES

- It is a modified sweat gland, present in pectoral region, retromammary space allows mobility
- 75% lymph nodes drain in axillary group, 20% in parasternal group and 5% in intercostal group
- Main support of the gland is suspensory ligament of Cooper
- Metastasis of carcinoma mammary gland occurs along lymphatics.

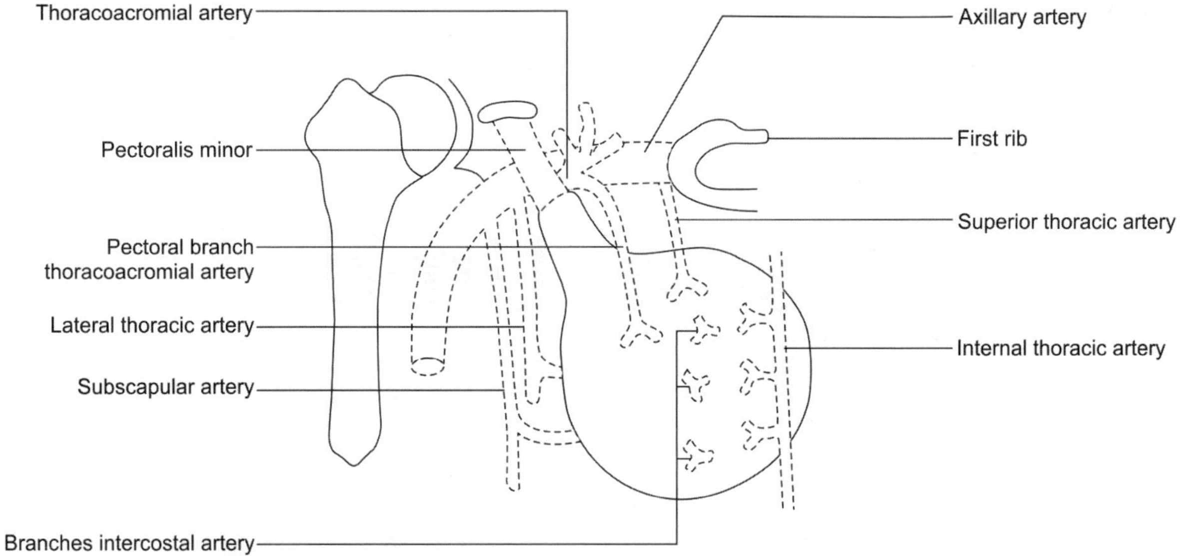

Figure 2.2: Mammary gland—blood supply (*For color version, see Plate 3*)

KEY FEATURES

- It is supplied by the branches of axillary, internal thoracic and intercostal arteries.

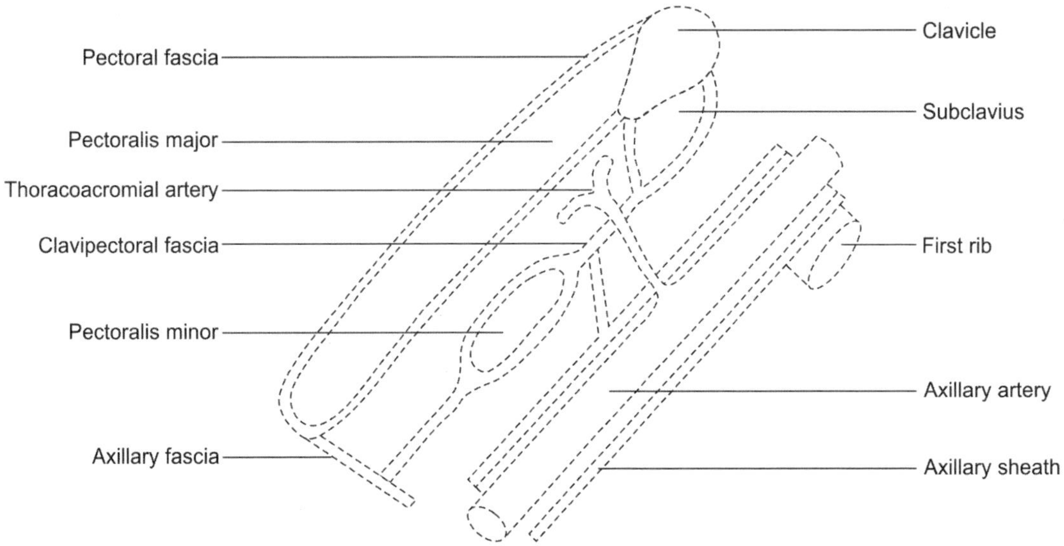

Figure 2.3: Clavipectoral fascia (*For color version, see Plate 4*)

KEY FEATURES

- It stretches between clavicle and pectoralis minor
- Above it splits to enclose subclavius and below it encloses pectoralis minor
- Laterally gets attached to coracoid process
- Following structures pierce the fascia:
  - Cephalic vein
  - Lateral pectoral nerve
  - Thoracoacromial artery
  - Lymphatics
- It covers 1st part of axillary artery.

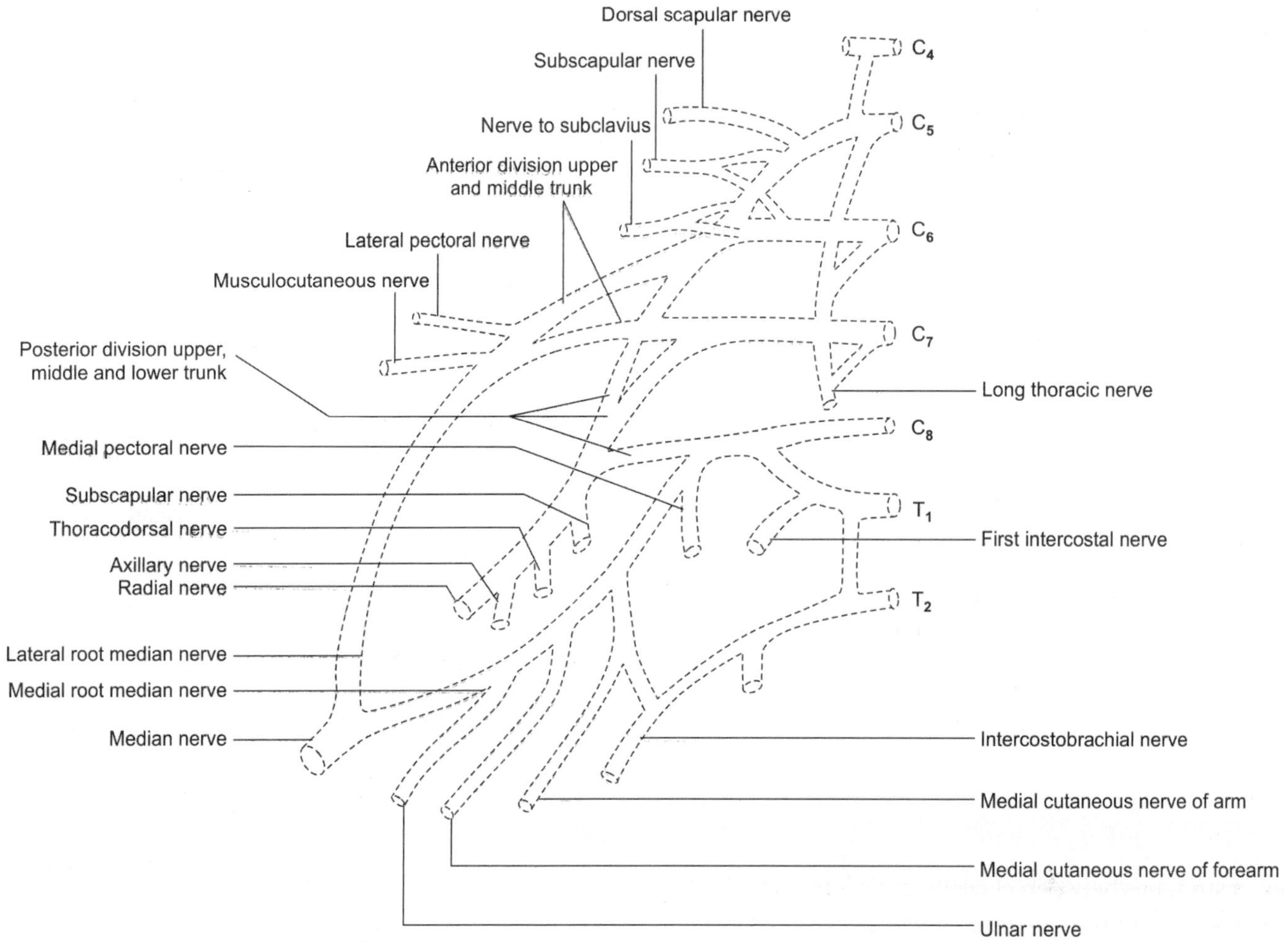

Figure 2.4: Brachial plexus (*For color version, see Plate 4*)

KEY FEATURES

- Formed by ventral rami C5678 and T1 spinal nerves
- Two nerves have complete root value radial and median (C5678 and T1)
- Erb's point—where six nerves unite; 2 roots (C56), 2 divisions of upper trunk and 2 nerves (suprascapular and nerve to subclavius). Injury at this point causes Erb's palsy
- Injury at the junction of C8 T1 causes Klumpke's palsy leading to claw hand
- Injury to long thoracic nerve causes winging of scapula.

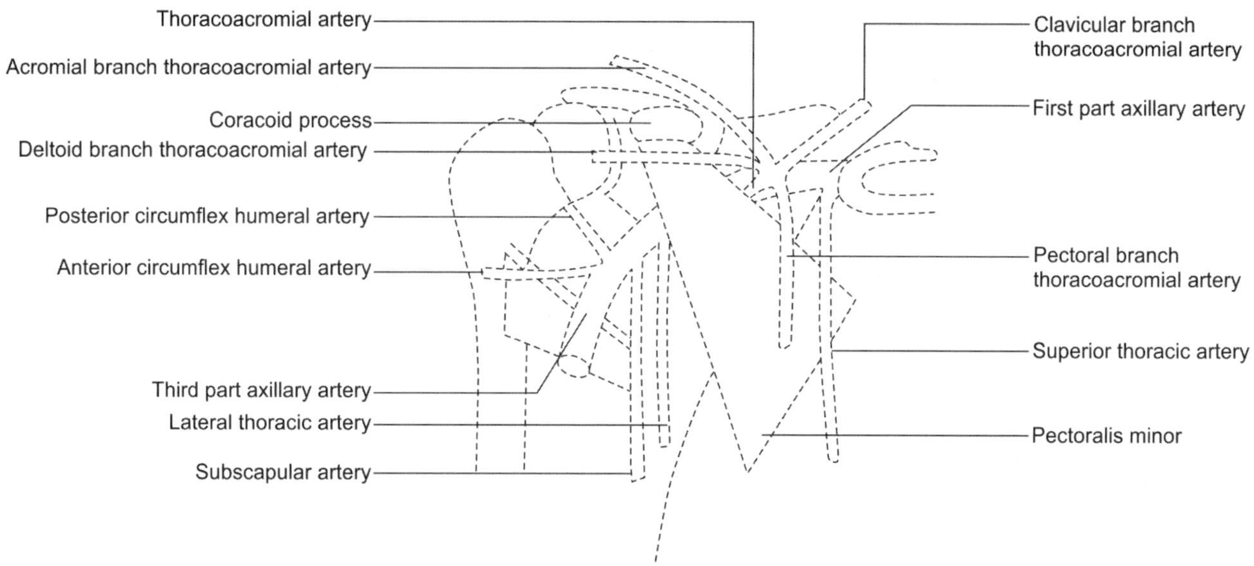

Figure 2.5: Axillary artery—branches

KEY FEATURES

- Axillary artery begins at the outer border of 1st rib and ends at lower border of teres major
- It is divided into three parts by pectoralis minor
- It is intimately related to brachial plexus in axilla
- 1st part—medial cord posteriorly, lateral and posterior cord laterally
- 2nd part—each cord in its respective direction as per the name (medial cord medially, lateral cord laterally and medial cord medial to axillary artery)
- 3rd part—branches of each cord will lie in their respective direction.

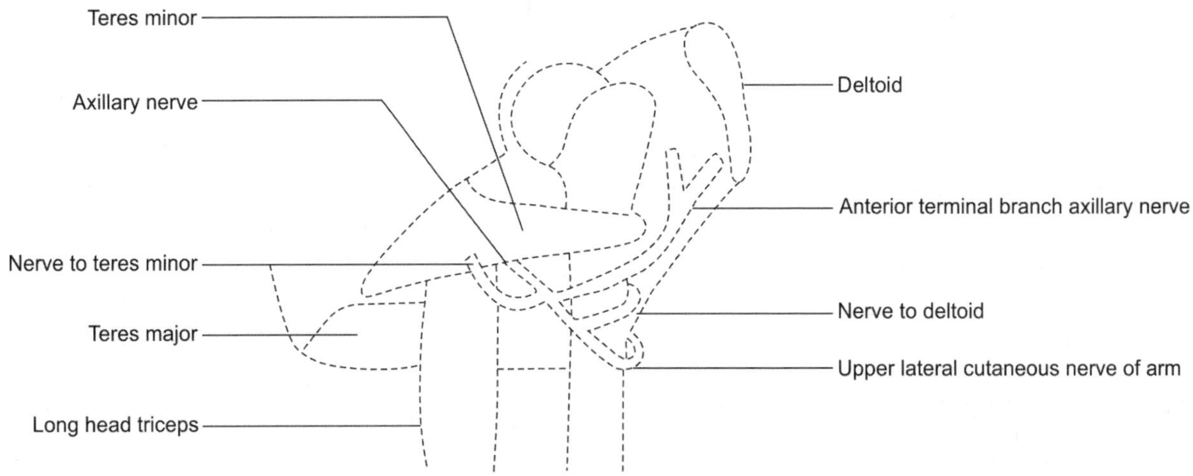

Figure 2.6: Axillary nerve—branches

KEY FEATURES

- Root value C56
- Leaves axilla with posterior circumflex humeral artery through upper quadrangular space
- It supplies deltoid and teres minor
- In fractured surgical neck humerus, it can be damaged leading to paralysis of deltoid.

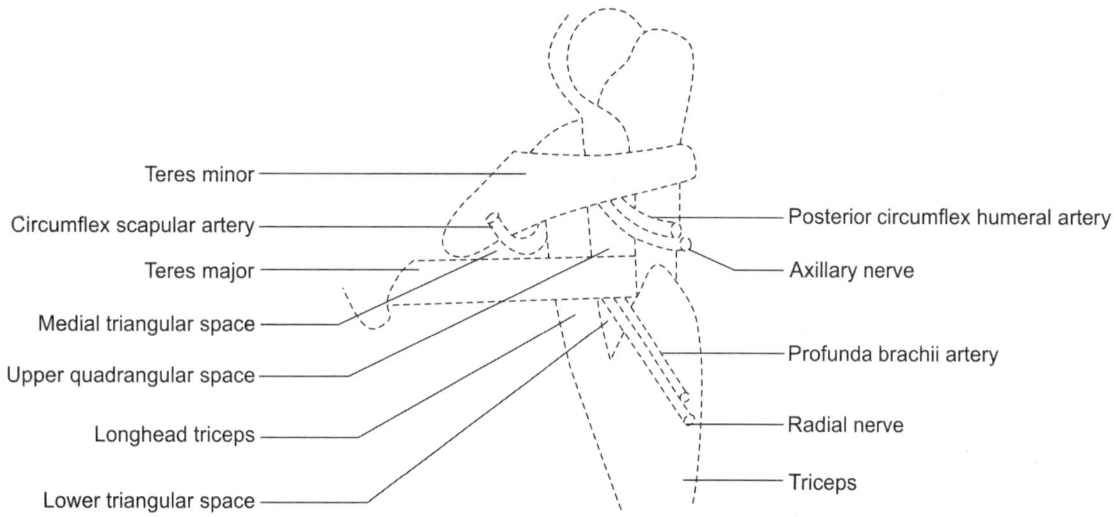

Figure 2.7: Spaces in scapular region

KEY FEATURES

- There are three spaces—two upper and one lower
- Upper medial space is triangular and circumflex scapular artery passes through it
- Upper lateral space is quadrangular and axillary nerve along with posterior circumflex humeral artery pass through it
- Lower triangular space allows the passage of radial nerve and profunda brachii artery.

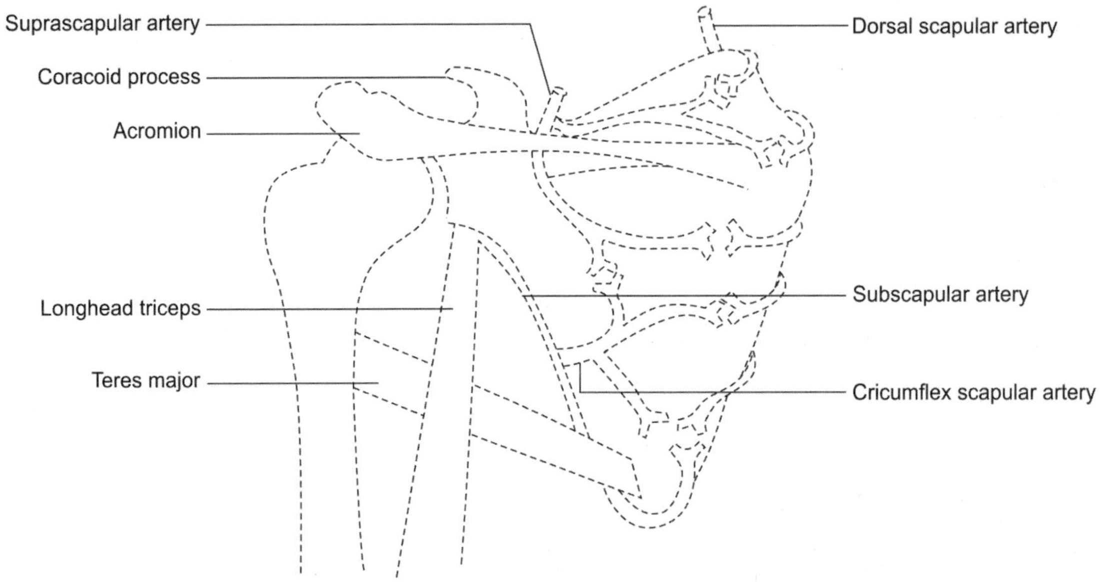

Figure 2.8: Anastomosis around scapula

KEY FEATURES

- Scapula is subjected to various movements due to the movements of free upper limb
- Therefore, it requires a rich anastomosis so that the blood supply is not compromised
- This anastomosis is formed by:
    - Suprascapular artery.
    - Dorsal scapular artery.
    - Circumflex scapular artery.

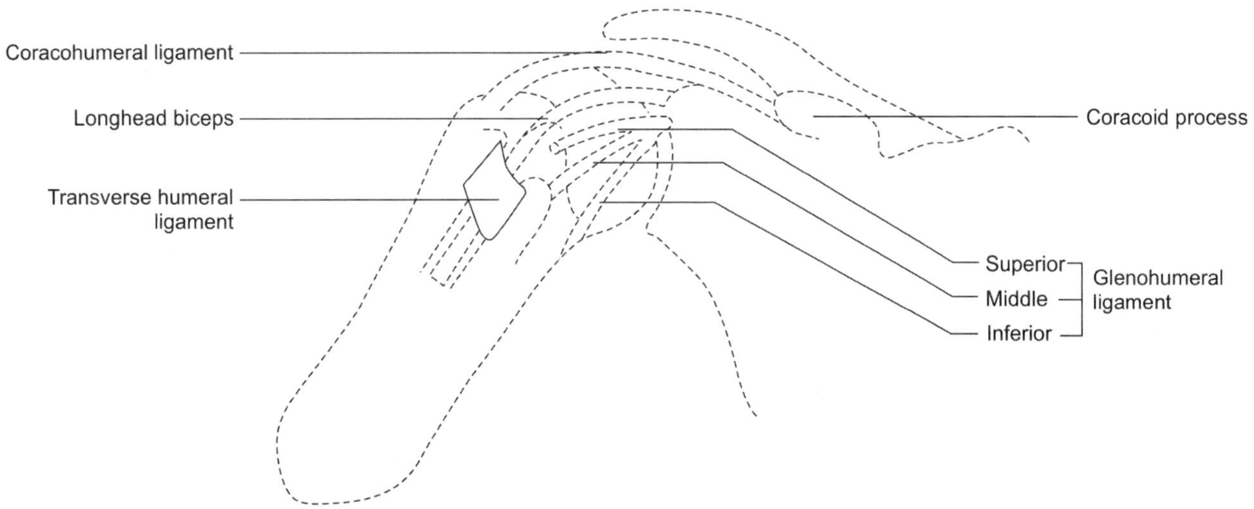

Figure 2.9: Shoulder joint

KEY FEATURES

- Factors which strengthen the shoulder joint are:
  - Rotator cuff which comprises of:
    - Subscapularis
    - Supraspinatus
    - Infraspinatus
    - Teres minor.
  - Coracohumeral ligament
  - Glenohumeral ligament:
    - Superior part attached to upper end lesser tubercle
    - Middle part attached to lower part lesser tubercle
    - Inferior part attached to lower part neck humerus.
  - Long head biceps.

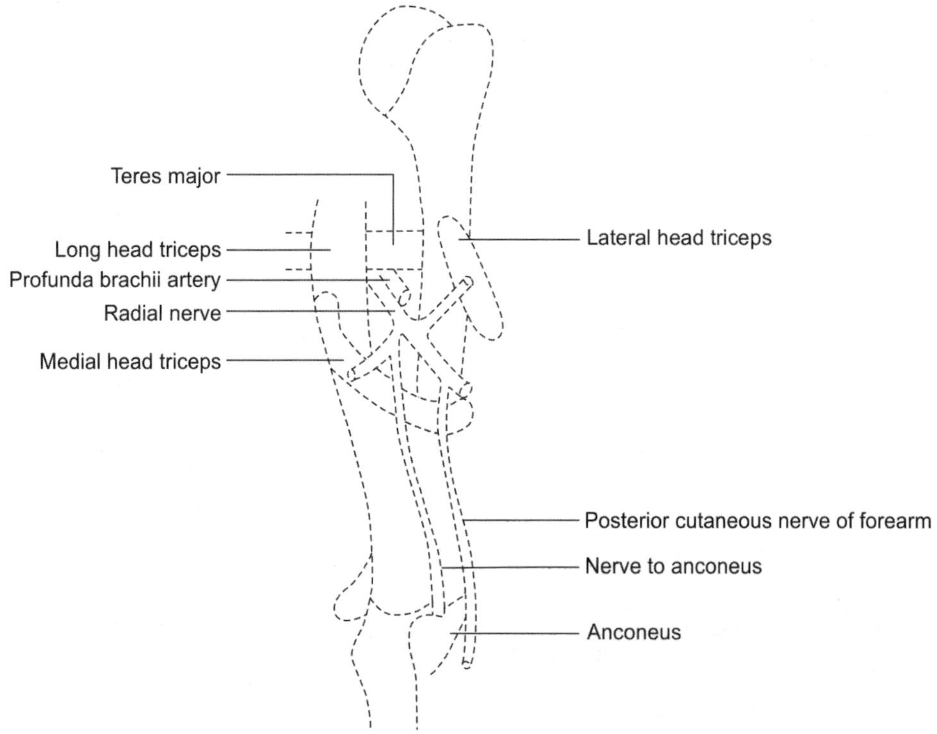

Figure 2.10: Radial nerve in radial groove

KEY FEATURES

- Accompanied by profunda brachii artery
- Runs between medial and lateral heads of triceps muscle and supplies them
- Nerve to medial head also supplies anconeus muscle
- Posterior cutaneous nerve of forearm arises from radial nerve before it leaves the groove
- Nerve leaves the radial groove by piercing lateral intermuscular septum at the junction of upper 2/3rd and lower 1/3rd of humerus
- Injury to the radial nerve in the groove paralyzes extensors of the wrist called wrist drop.

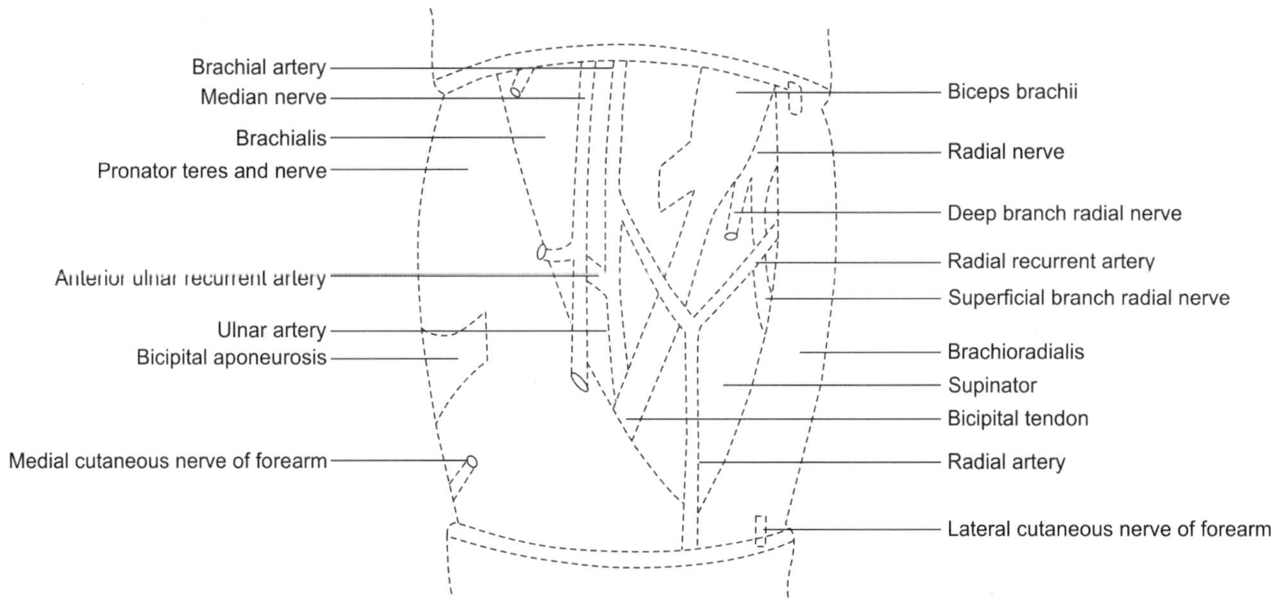

Figure 2.11: Cubital fossa

KEY FEATURES

- Roof formed by:
  - Skin, superficial fascia, medial and lateral cutaneous nerves of forearm
  - Median cubital vein resting on bicipital aponeurosis
  - Deep fascia of forearm
- Floor formed by—brachialis medially and supinator laterally
- Medial boundary—pronator teres
- Lateral boundary—brachioradialis
- Base—arbitrary line uniting medial and lateral epicondyles of humerus
- Apex—distally at the junction of medial and lateral walls.
- Contents—medial to lateral
  - Median nerve
  - Brachial artery and branches
  - Tendon of biceps
  - Radial nerve.

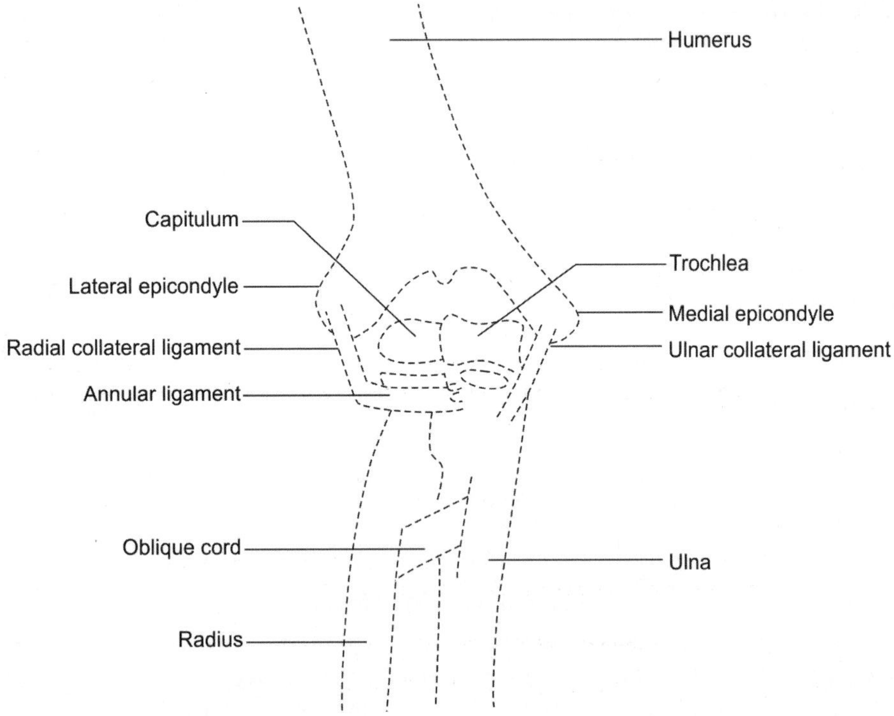

Figure 2.12: Elbow joint—anterior view

KEY FEATURES

- It is a compound, synovial hinge variety of joint
- It has two components:
  - Humeroulnar joint
  - Humeroradial joint
- The joint capsule encloses superior radioulnar joint, hence collectively called cubital articulations
- A carrying angle is formed between the long axis of upper arm and forearm
- This angle is open laterally and is 163°.

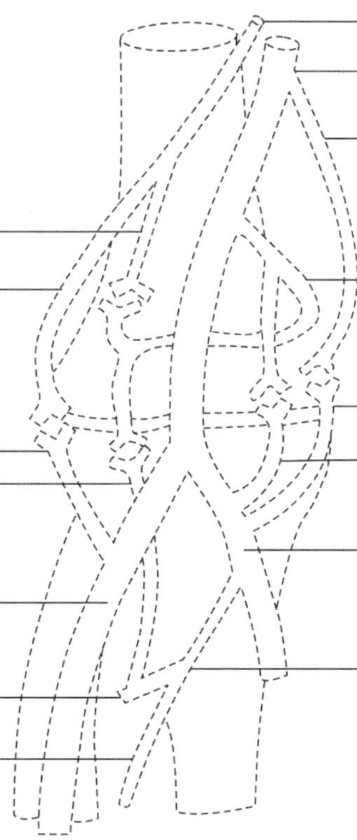

Figure 2.13: Anastomosis around elbow

KEY FEATURES

- It occurs between the branches of brachial artery and proximal parts of radial and ulnar arteries
- During flexion of the elbow the brachial artery is likely to be kinked leading to sluggish blood flow, thus cubital anastomosis is essential.

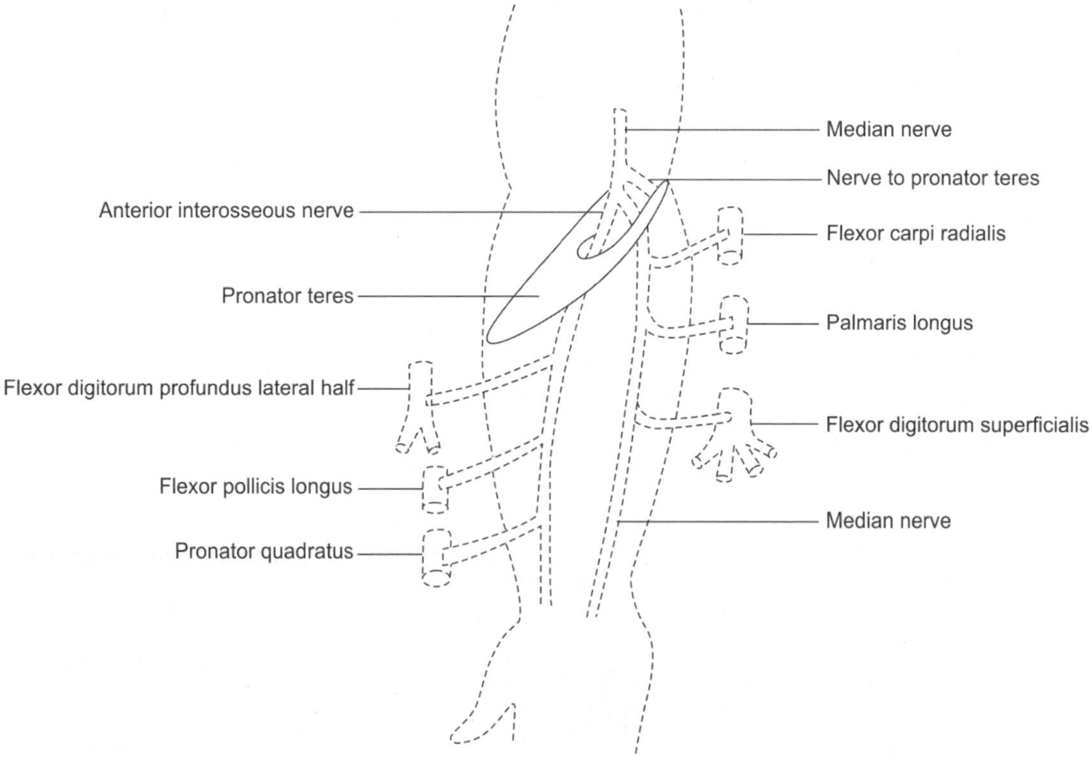

Figure 2.14: Median nerve in forearm

KEY FEATURES

- In cubital fossa it gives a branch to pronator teres and then passes between two heads of pronator teres to enter forearm
- It supplies all muscles on the flexor aspect of forearm except flexor carpi ulnaris, medial half flexor digitorum profundus.

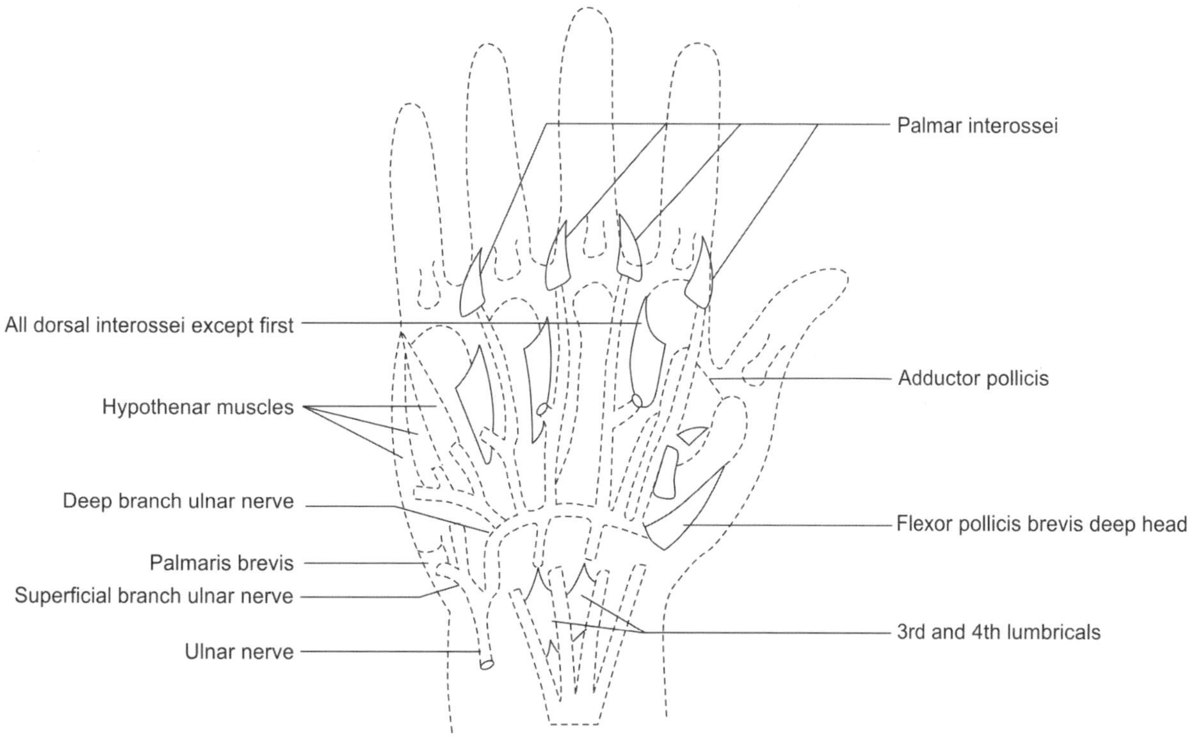

Figure 2.15: Ulnar nerve in hand

KEY FEATURES

- Ulnar nerve enters palm superficial to flexor retinaculum
- It supplies cutaneous branches to little finger and ulnar half ring finger
- It supplies all intrinsic muscles of palm except thenar eminence and 1st, 2nd lumbricals
- Its injury leads to claw hand.

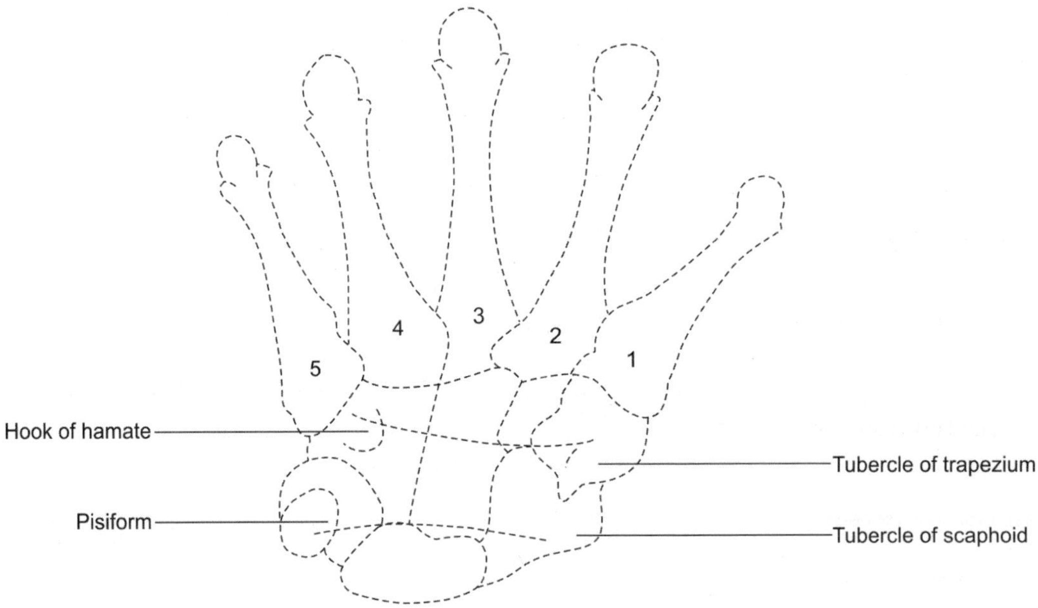

Figure 2.16: Flexor retinaculum

KEY FEATURES

- Flexor retinaculum along with carpals forms an osteofascial tunnel called carpal tunnel
- Through these tunnel long flexors of the digits and medial nerve enter palm
- Compression of median nerve due to dislocation of lunate gives rise to carpal tunnel syndrome
- This causes weakness and wasting of thenar muscles and loss of sensation in lateral three and half fingers.

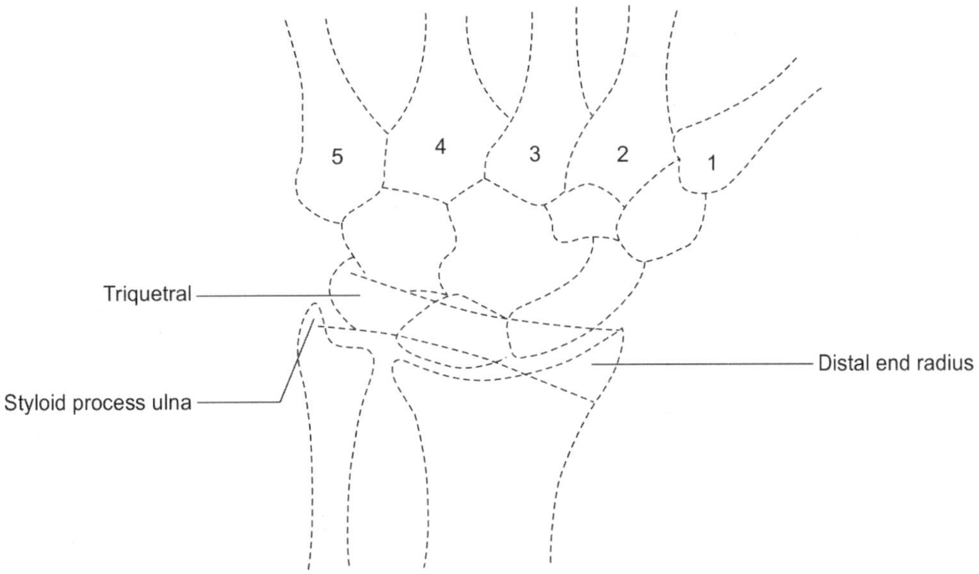

Figure 2.17: Extensor retinaculum

KEY FEATURES

- It allows the passage of tendons to digits through various compartments
- There are six compartments from lateral to medial side:
    i. Abductor pollicis longus and extensor pollicis brevis.
    ii. Extensor carpi radialis longus and brevis.
    iii. Extensor pollicis longus.
    iv. Extensor digitorum and indices.
    v. Extensor digiti minimi.
    vi. Extensor carpi ulnaris.

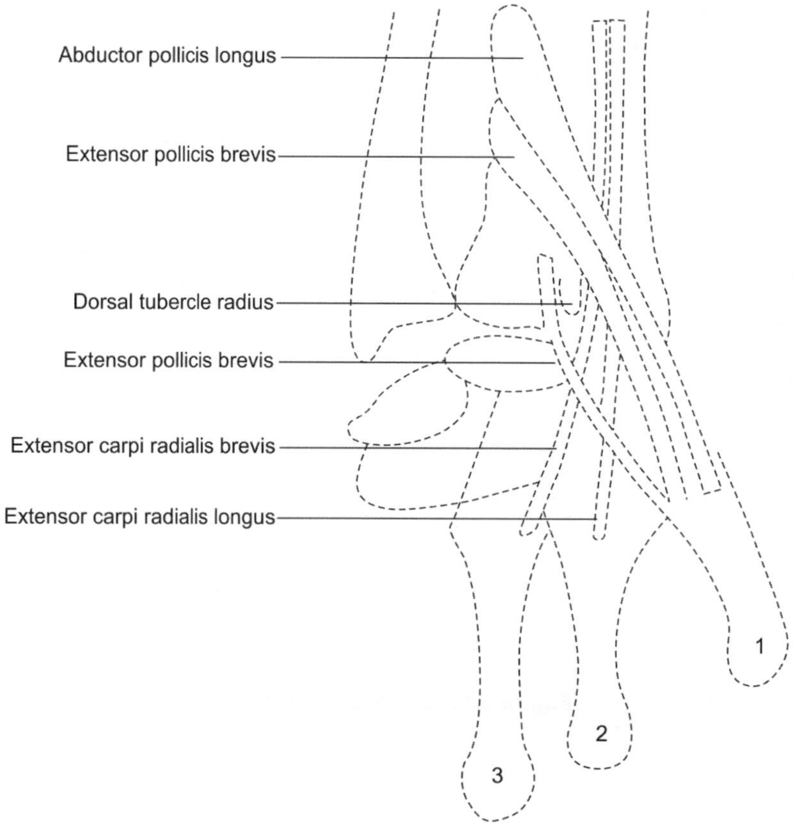

Figure 2.18: Anatomical snuff box

KEY FEATURES

- Laterally—abductor pollicis longus and extensor pollicis brevis
- Medially—extensor pollicis longus
- Roof—beginning of cephalic vein crossed by superficial branch radial nerve
- Floor—styloid process radius, scaphoid, trapezium, base of 1st metacarpal, extensor carpi radialis longus and brevis
- Content—radial artery
- In fractured neck scaphoid, pain occurs in anatomical snuff box on pressure.

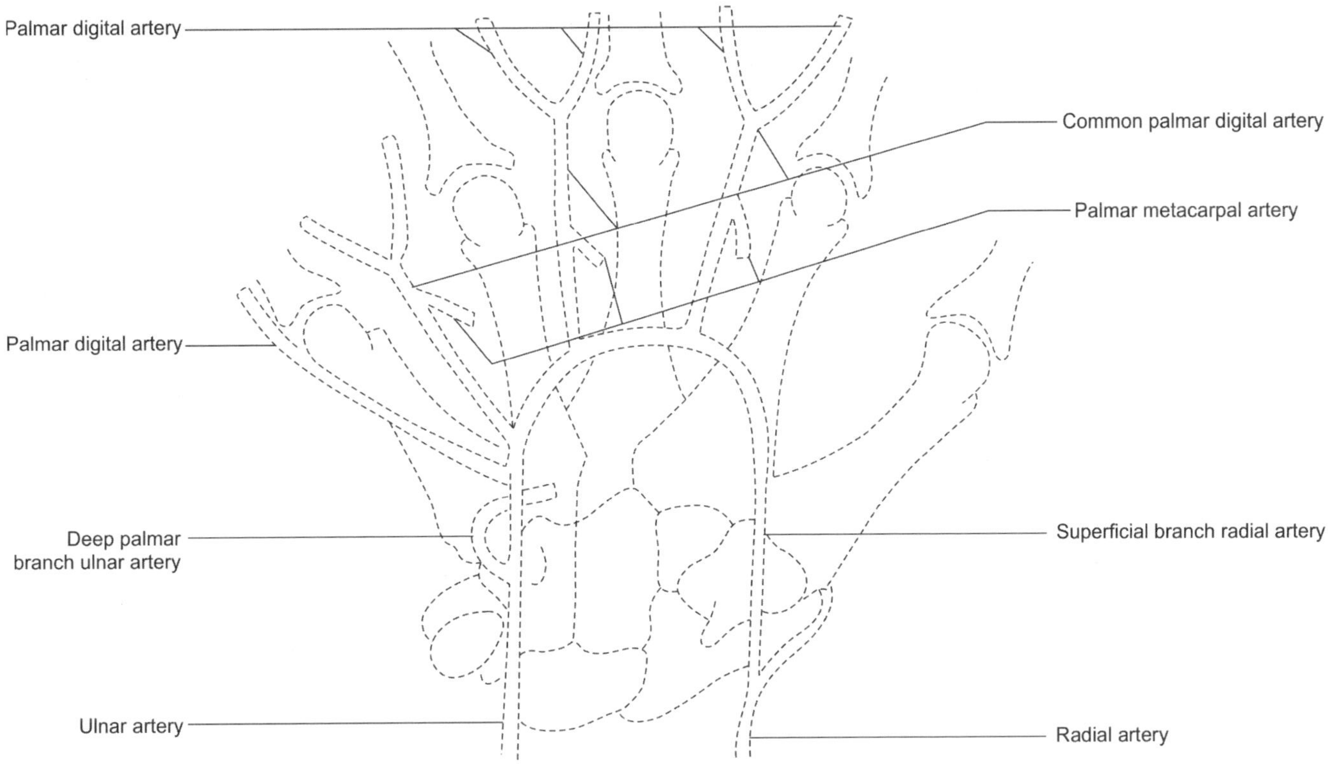

Figure 2.19: Superficial palmar arch

KEY FEATURES

- Formed mainly by ulnar artery present below palmar aponeurosis
- It may be completed by superficial branch radial artery
- Supplies palmar digital branches to medial three and half fingers
- Common palmar digital arteries anastomose with palmar metacarpal arteries.

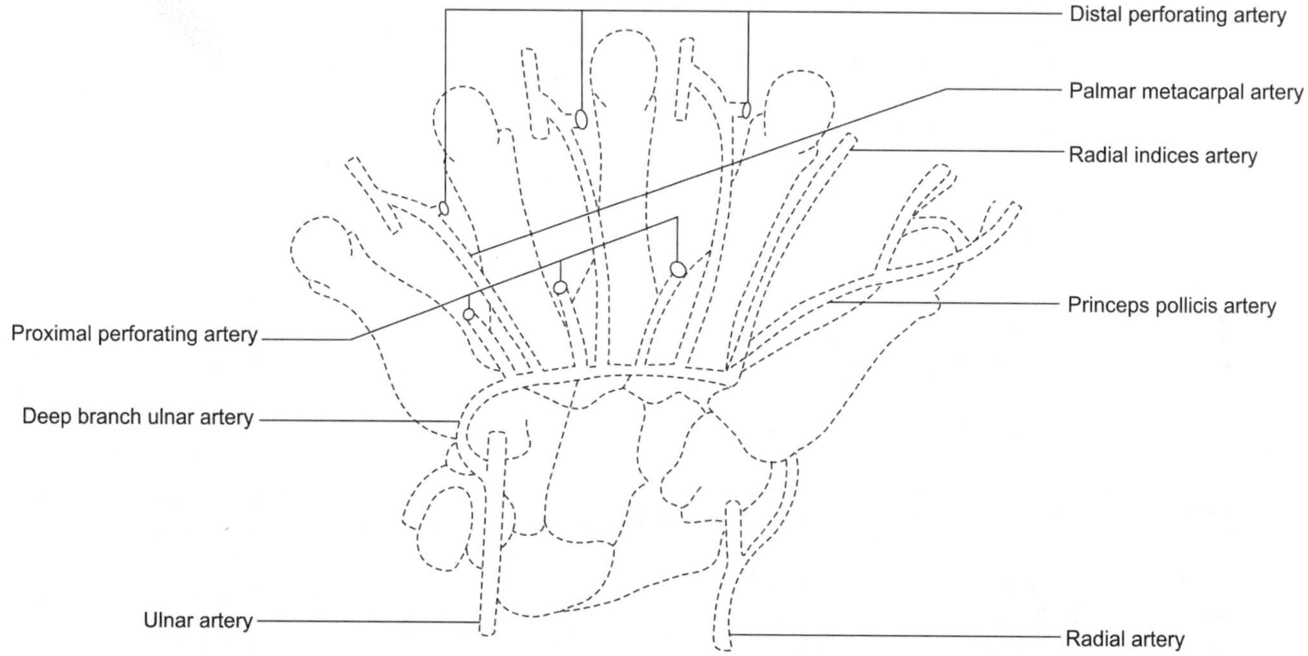

Figure 2.20: Deep palmar arch

KEY FEATURES

- Formed by the anastomosis of radial artery which enters palm through 1st interosseus space and deep branch of ulnar artery
- It supplies thumb and radial side index finger
- Three proximal perforators arise from the arch and enter dorsum of hand through proximal part of 2,3,4 interosseus spaces
- Three distal perforators arising from three palmar metacarpal arteries enter dorsum of hand through distal part of 2,3,4 interosseus spaces.

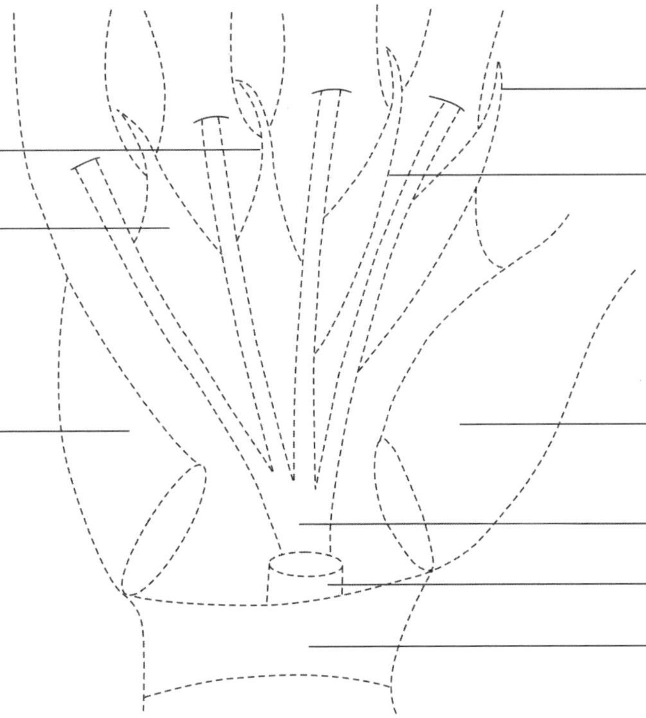

Figure 2.21: Lumbricals

KEY FEATURES

- Four in number, 1st and 2nd are unipennate, 3rd and 4th are bipennate
- They arise from the tendons of flexor digitorum profundus
- 1st and 2nd lumbricals are supplied by median nerve whereas 3rd and 4th are supplied by ulnar nerve
- Action—they flex metacarpophalangeal joints and extend interphalangeal joints.

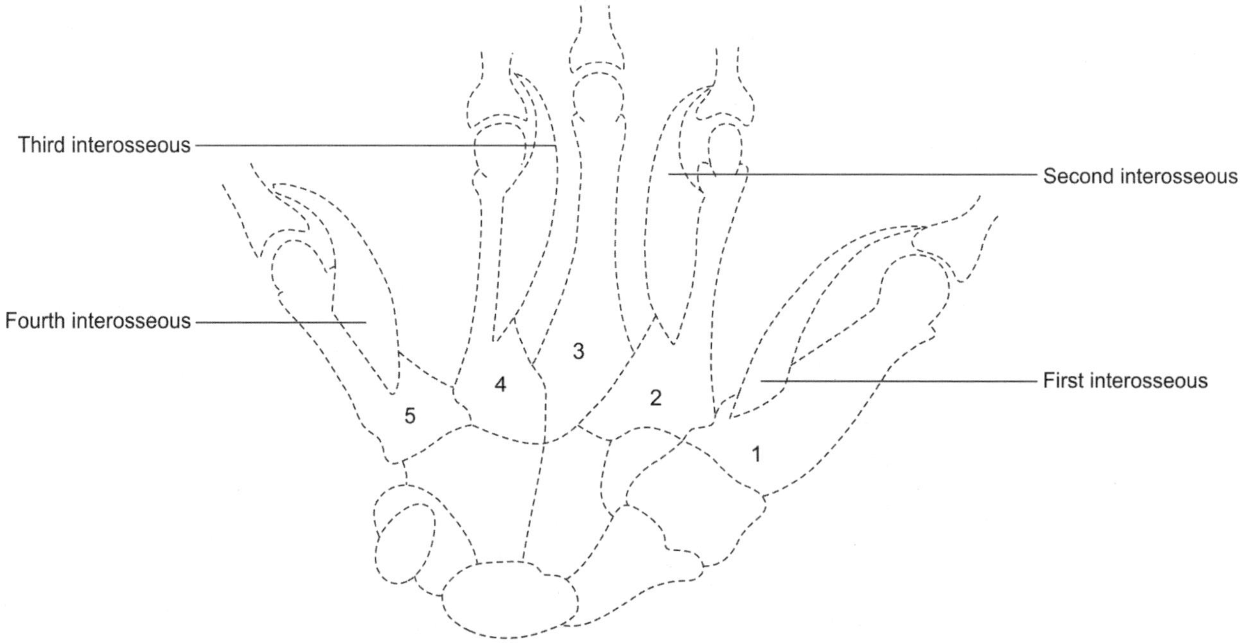

Figure 2.22: Palmar interossei (right hand)

KEY FEATURES

- Four in number and unipennate
- Middle finger acts as central axis of movement hence does not have any interosseous
- Action—they are adductors of fingers.

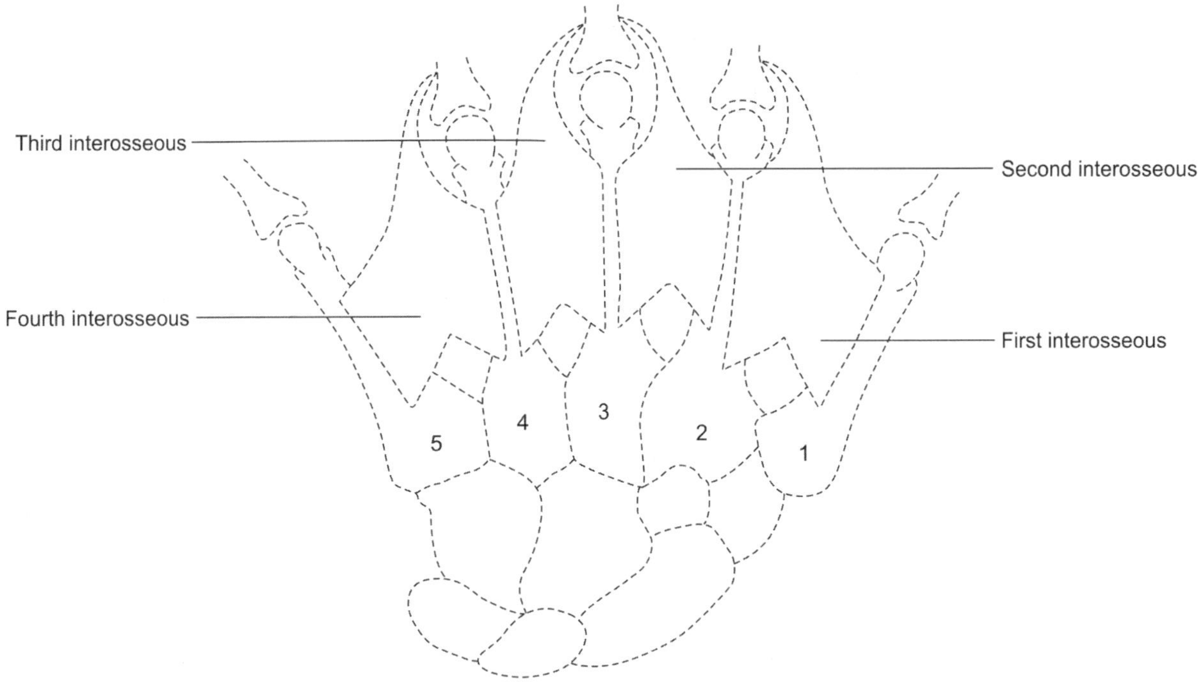

Figure 2.23: Dorsal interossei (left hand)

KEY FEATURES

- Four in number and bipennate
- Middle finger receives two dorsal interossei
- Action—they are abductors of fingers.

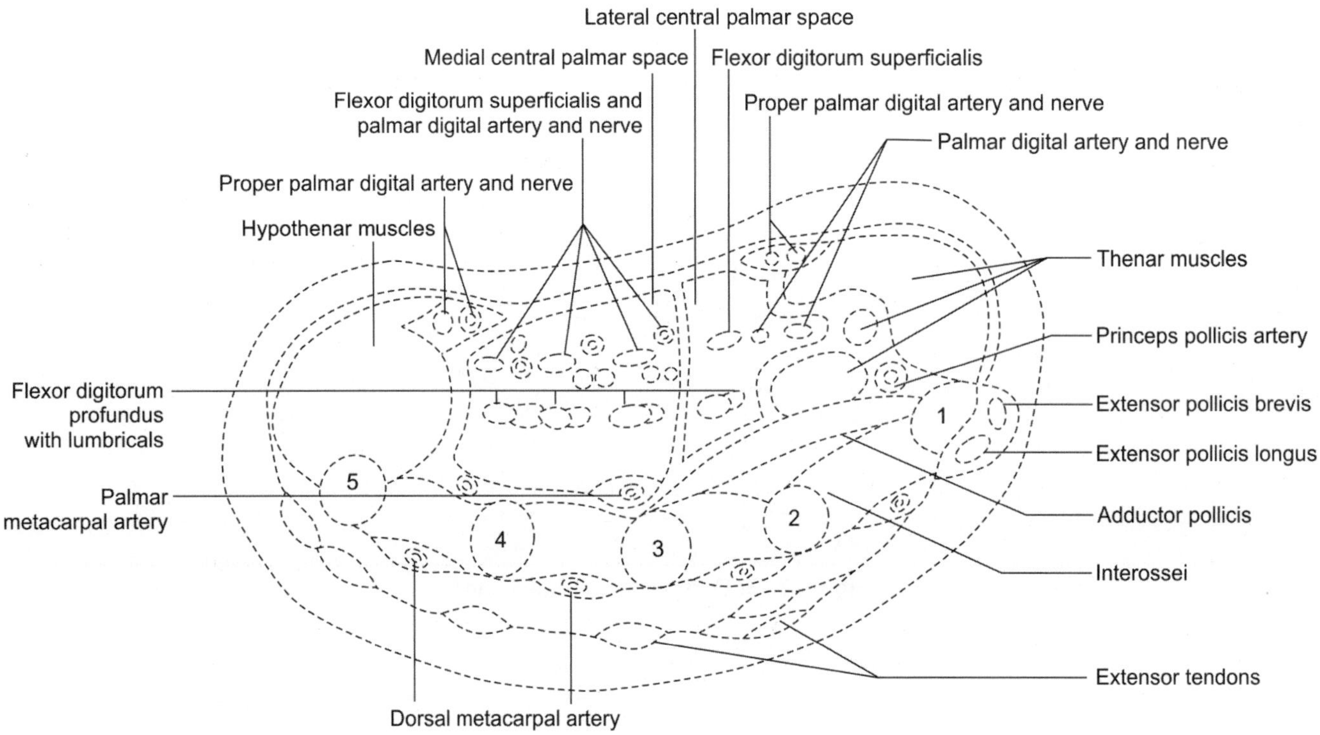

Figure 2.24: Palmar spaces

KEY FEATURES

- There are four palmar spaces
- Hypothenar space encloses small muscles of little finger (hypothenar muscles)
- Thenar space encloses small muscles of thumb (thenar muscles)
- The central part of the palm is divided into two spaces by a septum which extends between palmar aponeurosis and shaft 3rd metacarpal into medial and lateral central palmar spaces
- These central spaces continue distally as lumbrical canals
- The pus can be drained through respective webs of fingers.

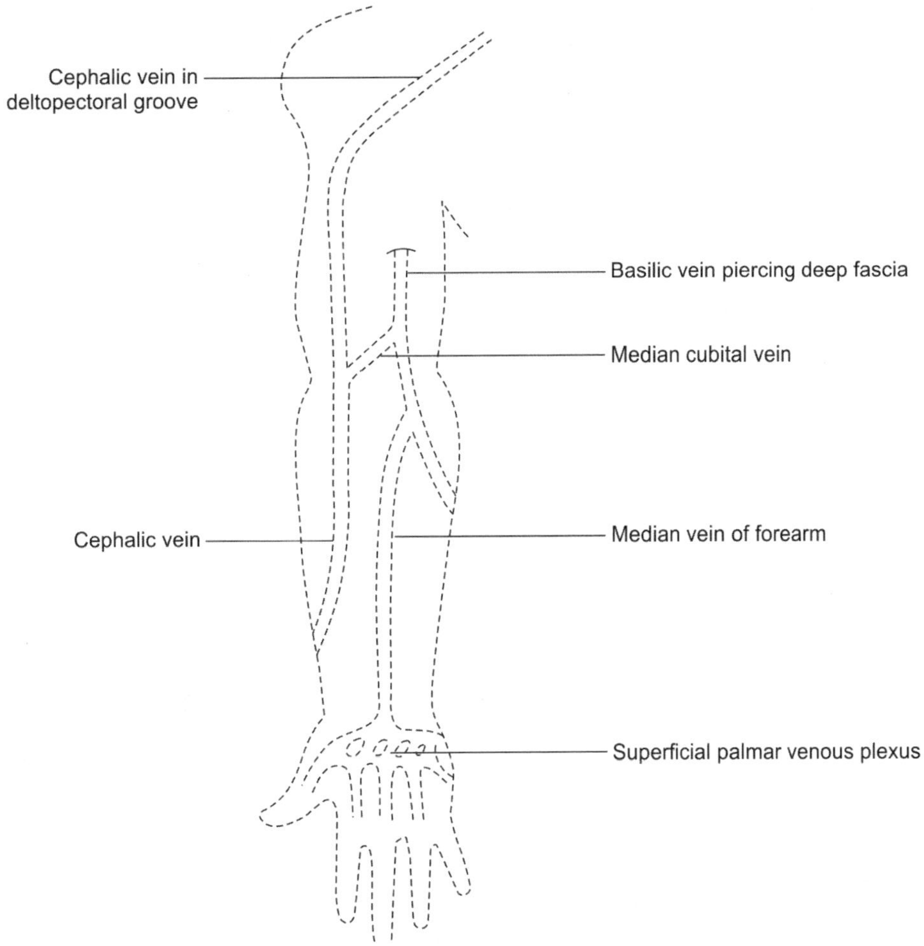

Figure 2.25: Venous drainage

KEY FEATURES

- Cephalic vein drains the lateral side of upper limb, passes through deltopectoral groove, then pierces clavipectoral fascia to end in axillary vein
- Basilic vein drains the medial side of upper limb, median vein of forearm drains into it
- This vein pierces deep fascia in the middle of upper arm and opens into axillary vein
- In front of the bicipital aponeurosis cephalic and basilic veins are interconnected by median cubital vein
- Cannulation through basilic vein for cardiac catheterization is preferable because of its continuity with axillary vein without angulation
- Median cubital vein is used for I/V injections and transfusions.

CHAPTER 3

Head and Neck

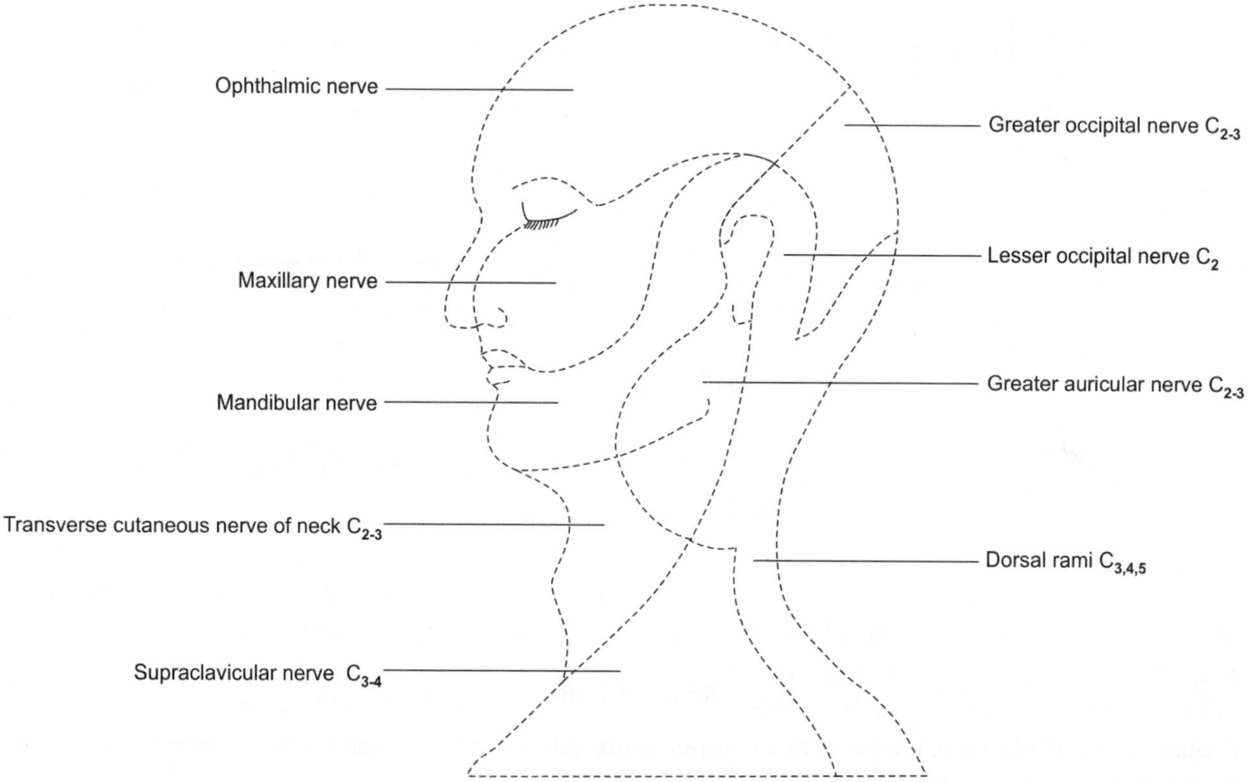

Figure 3.1: Dermatomes (*For color version, see Plate 5*)

KEY FEATURES

- The cutaneous nerve supply of face and part of head is unique as compared to rest of the body
- It is supplied by three divisions of trigeminal nerve, namely ophthalmic, maxillary and mandibular
- Rest of the area is supplied by $C_{2,3,4}$ spinal segments
- 1st spinal nerve does not have any dermatome
- Skin over the angle of the mandible is supplied by C_2.

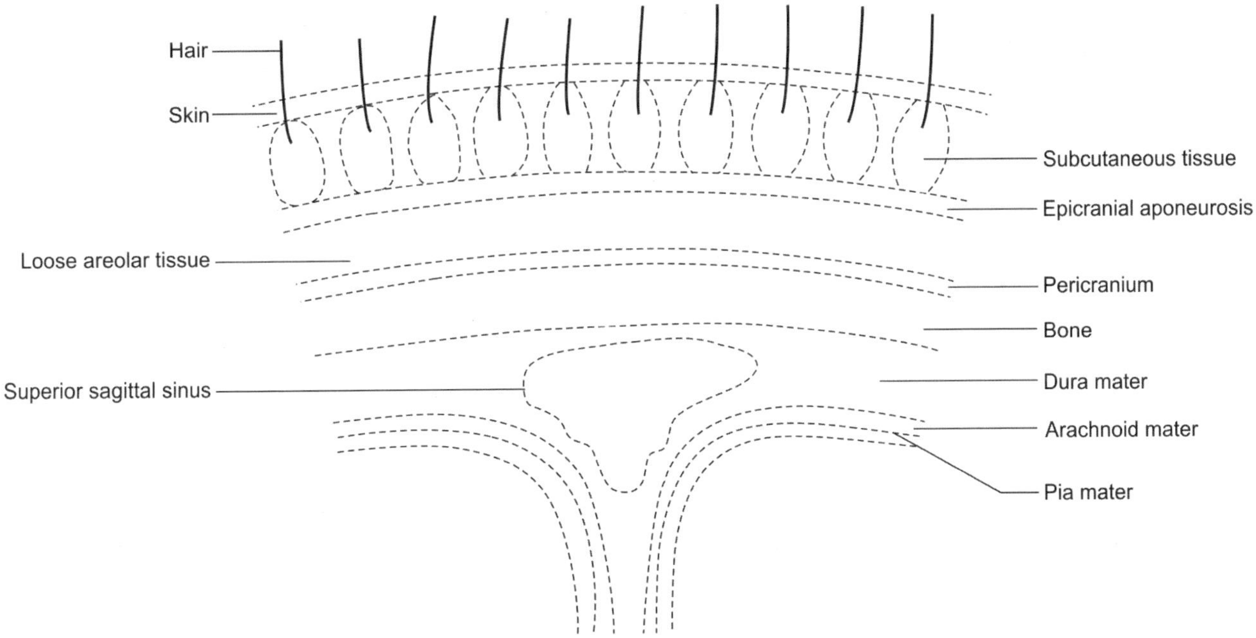

Figure 3.2: Layers of scalp (*For color version, see Plate 5*)

KEY FEATURES

- Skin, subcutaneous tissue and epicranial aponeurosis moves as a unit because they are bound by connective tissue septa
- The walls of the blood vessels are bound to the septa which prevent them to retract during injury. Thus, wounds of the scalp bleed profusely and can be stopped by applying pressure against bone
- If epicranial aponeurosis is cut the wound will gape
- Loose areolar tissue is the dangerous area of scalp because it is traversed by emissary veins
- Any collection of blood can give rise to black eye because frontalis has no bony attachment.

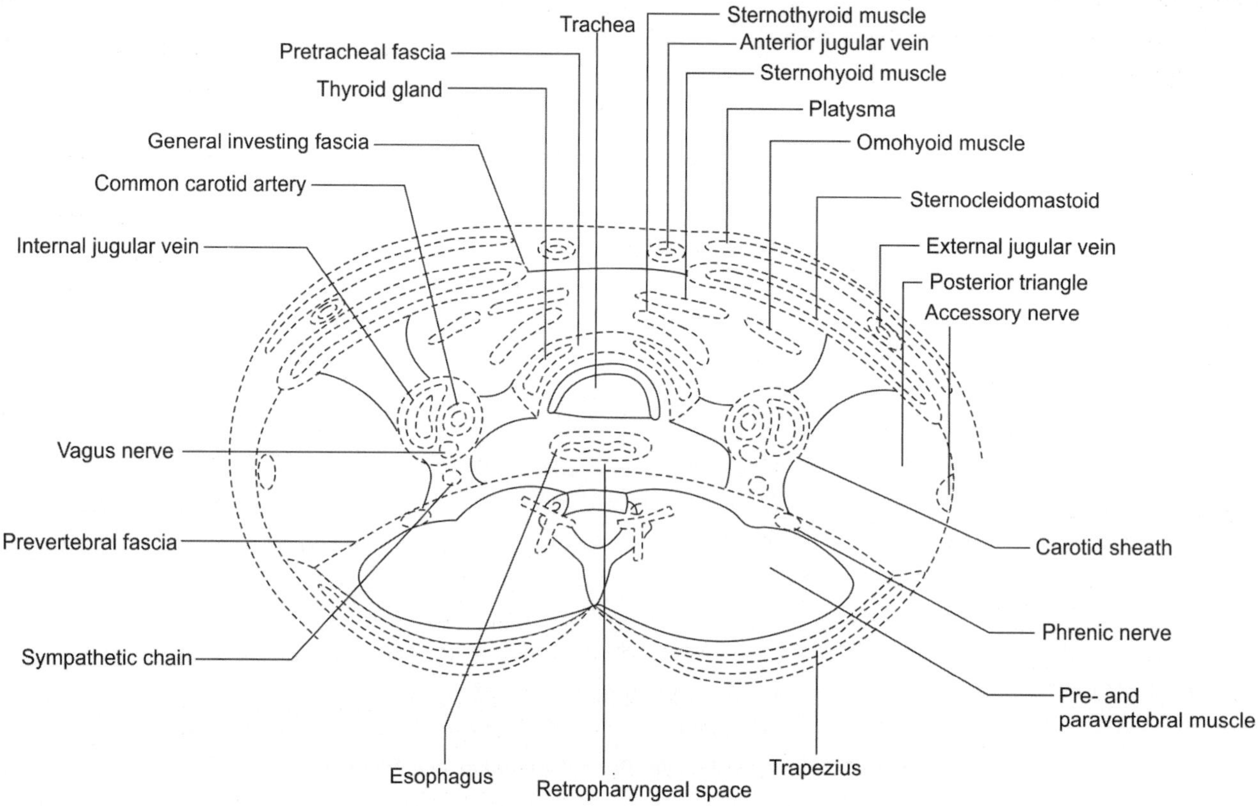

Figure 3.3: Deep cervical fascia—level C_7 (*For color version, see Plate 6*)

KEY FEATURES

- It has three components:
  i. General investing—encloses neck in the form of a sleeve. It encloses two muscles (sternocleidomastoid, trapezius), two glands (parotid, submandibular) and two spaces (supraclavicular, suprasternal).
  ii. Prevertebral—covers prevertebral muscles and forms the floor of posterior triangle of neck.
  iii. Pretracheal—encloses thyroid gland and is attached to hyoid to form ligament of Berry.
- All the three components contribute to the formation of a sheath around the neurovascular bundle of neck called carotid sheath. It extends from root of neck to the base of skull
- It encloses—common and internal carotid arteries, internal jugular vein and vagus nerve. In its walls there are embedded roots of ansa cervicalis.

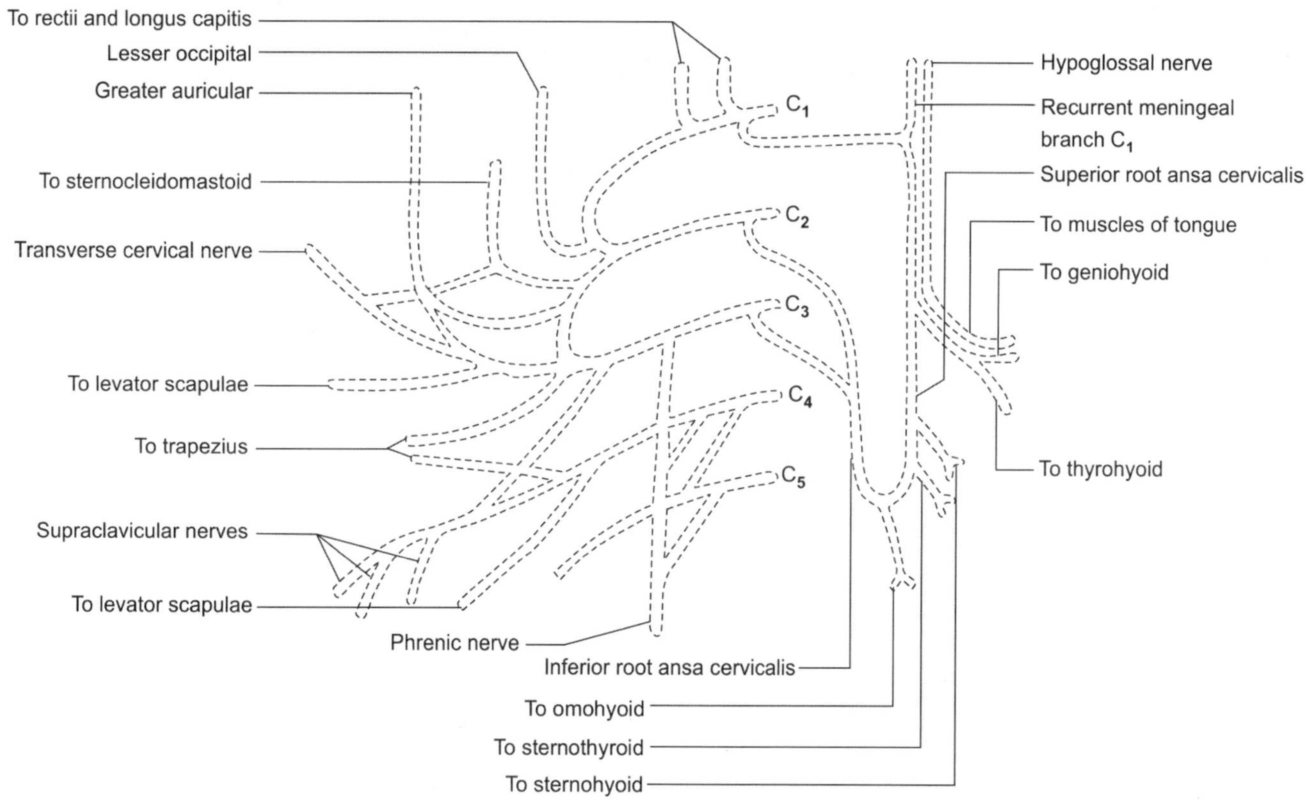

Figure 3.4: Cervical plexus (*For color version, see Plate 6*)

KEY FEATURES

- C_1 is purely motor and has no dermatome. Some fibers join and run in the sheath of hypoglossal nerve and in carotid triangle separate from 12th nerve to form superior root of ansa cervicalis and supplies geniohyoid, thyrohyoid
- $C_{2,3}$ join to form inferior root of ansa cervicalis. Both the roots are embedded in carotid sheath. Ansa cervicalis supplies omohyoid, sternohyoid and sternothyroid
- $C_{2,3,4}$ supplies proprioceptive fibers to trapezius and sternocliedomastoid
- $C_{3,4,5}$ combine to form phrenic nerve which supplies diaphragm. It also forms supraclavicular nerves.

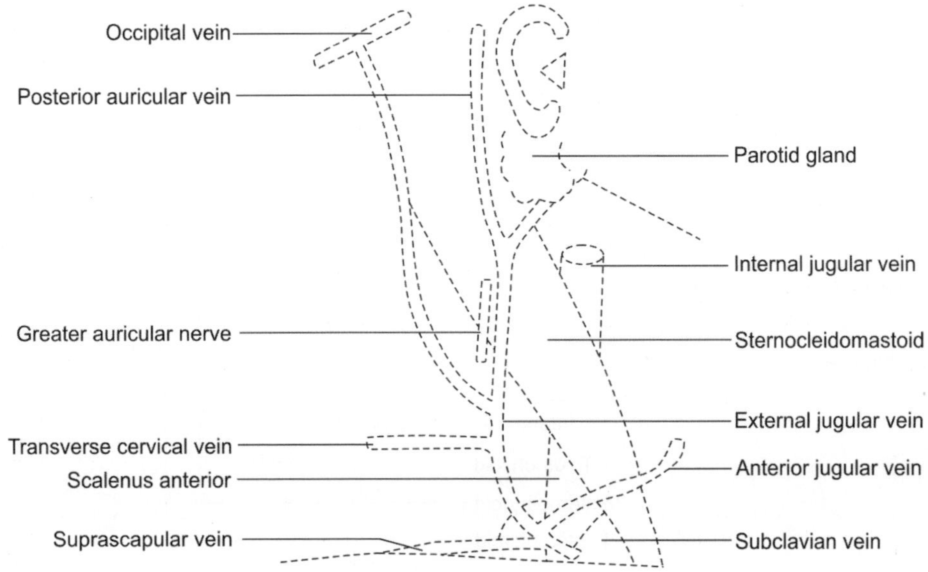

Figure 3.5: External jugular vein

KEY FEATURES

- It is formed by the union of posterior auricular vein and posterior division of retromandibular vein just below the angle of mandible
- It runs down and pierces the investing layer of deep fascia 2.5 cm above clavicle to enter supraclavicular triangle and terminates in subclavian vein
- The adventitia of external jugular vein merges with investing layer of deep fascia, thus preventing the vein to retract in case of injury and may cause air embolism.

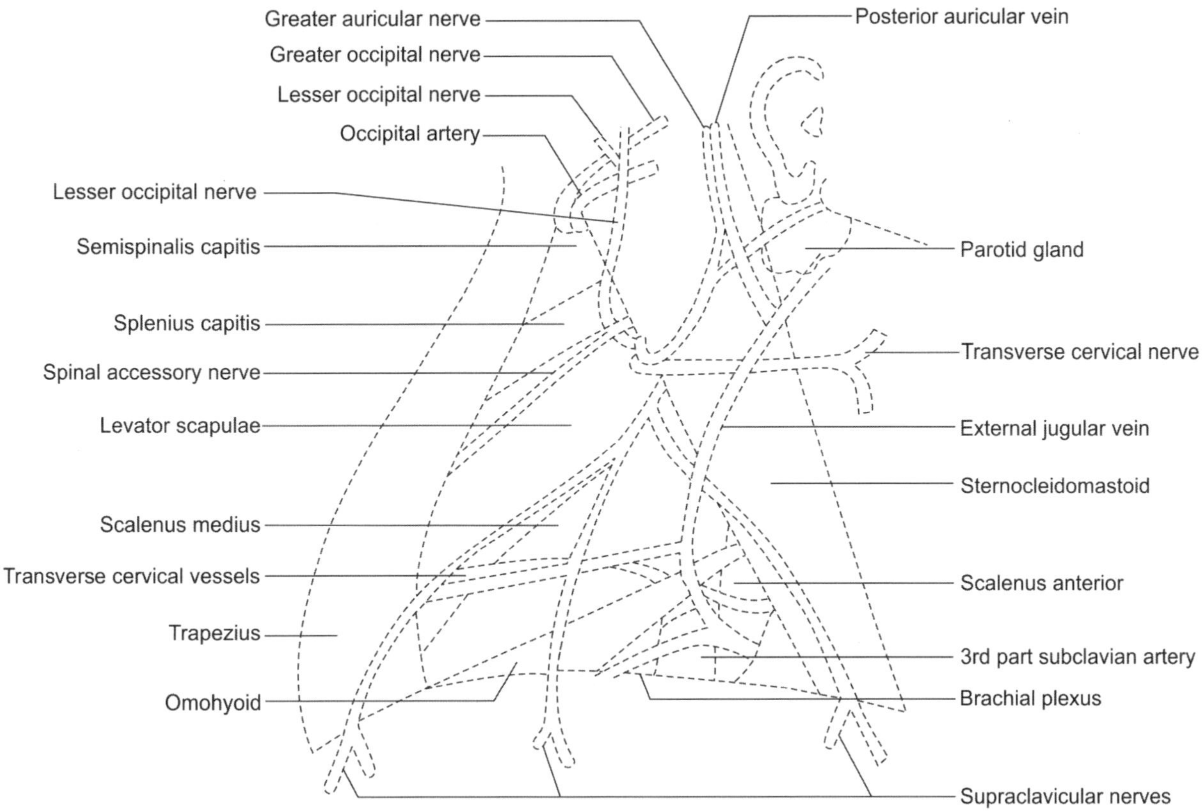

Figure 3.6: Posterior triangle of neck

KEY FEATURES

- Apex, anterior and posterior boundaries are formed by muscles (sternocleidomastoid and trapezius)
- Base is formed by bone (middle 1/3rd clavicle)
- Floor and roof are formed by fascia (prevertebral and general investing)
- Roof is pierced by—lesser occipital, greater auricular, transverse cervical and supraclavicular nerves, external jugular vein
- True content—spinal accessory nerve
- 3rd part subclavian artery and cervical part brachial plexus lie behind prevertebral fascia.

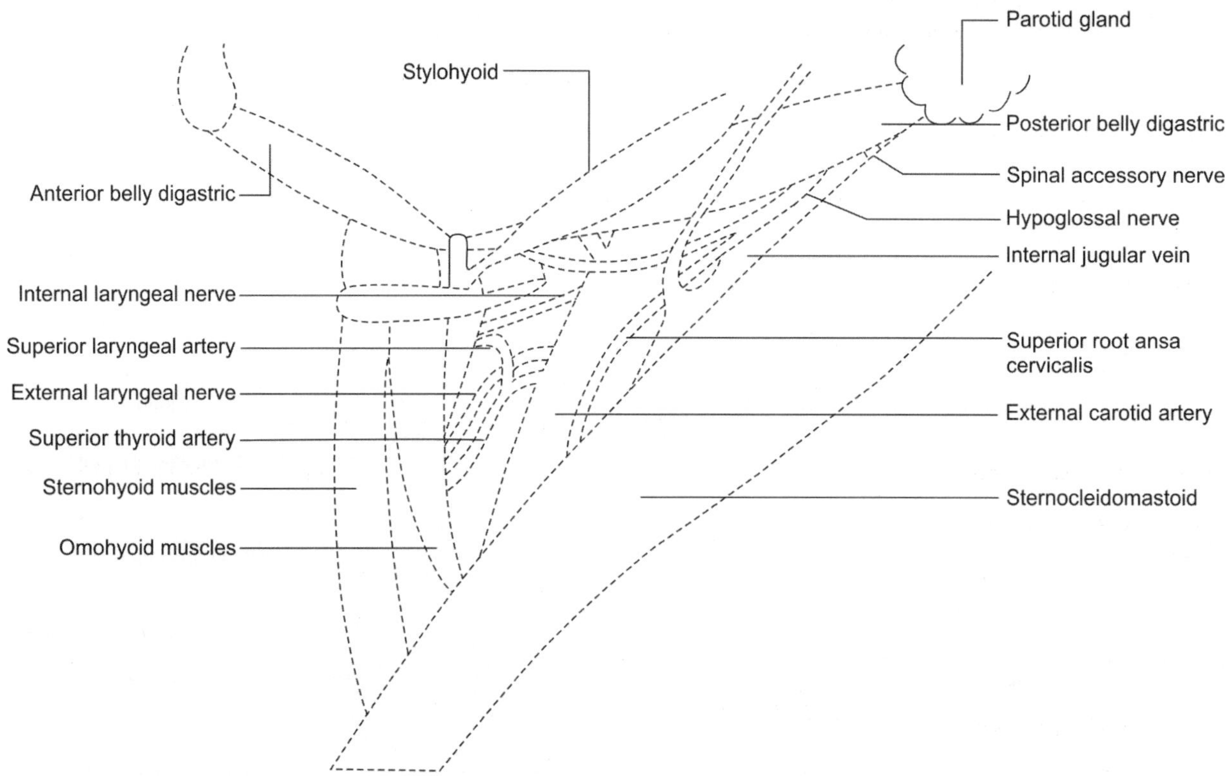

Figure 3.7: Carotid triangle

KEY FEATURES

- Boundaries:
  - Superiorly—posterior belly digastric, stylohyoid
  - Posteriorly—anterior border sternocleidomastoid
  - Anteroinferiorly—superior belly omohyoid
- Roof: Investing layer of deep fascia, platysma, cervical branch facial nerve, transverse cervical nerve
- Floor: Above downwards—Hyoglossus lower part, thyrohyoid, middle and inferior constrictor
- Contents: External carotid artery and its branches, hypoglossal and spinal accessory nerves, ansa cervicalis, external and internal laryngeal nerves
- Carotid sheath and its contents lie behind sternocleidomastoid muscle. Common carotid artery can be palpated 4 cm above sternoclavicular joint by pressing against carotid tubercle of 6th cervical vertebra.

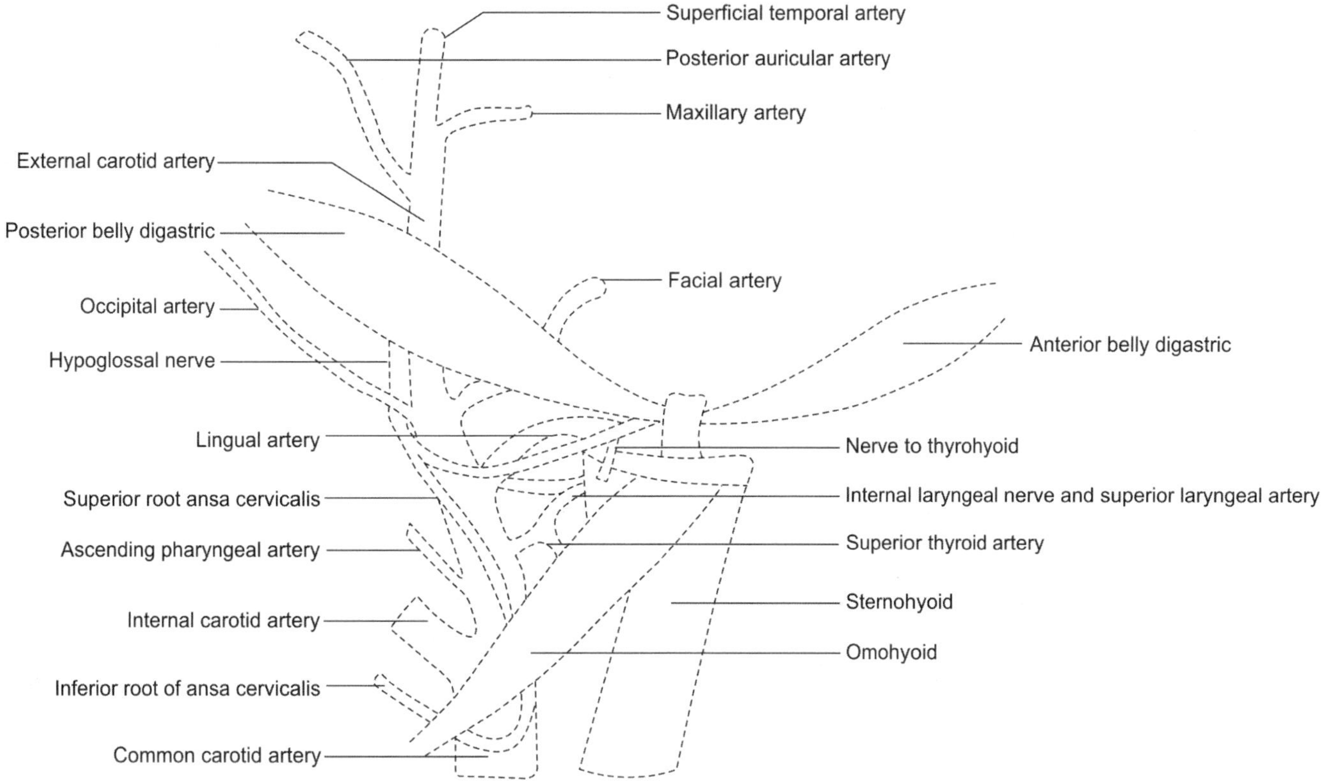

Figure 3.8: External carotid artery

KEY FEATURES

- Arises from common carotid at the level of upper border of thyroid cartilage
- It leaves the carotid sheath and gives off five branches in carotid triangle, namely—ascending pharyngeal, superior thyroid, lingual, facial and occipital arteries
- After leaving the triangle it gives off posterior auricular and two terminal branches—maxillary and superficial temporal arteries
- The lingual artery forms a loop over the greater cornu of the hyoid which is crossed laterally by hypoglossal nerve. This loop of the lingual artery permits free movement of hyoid bone.

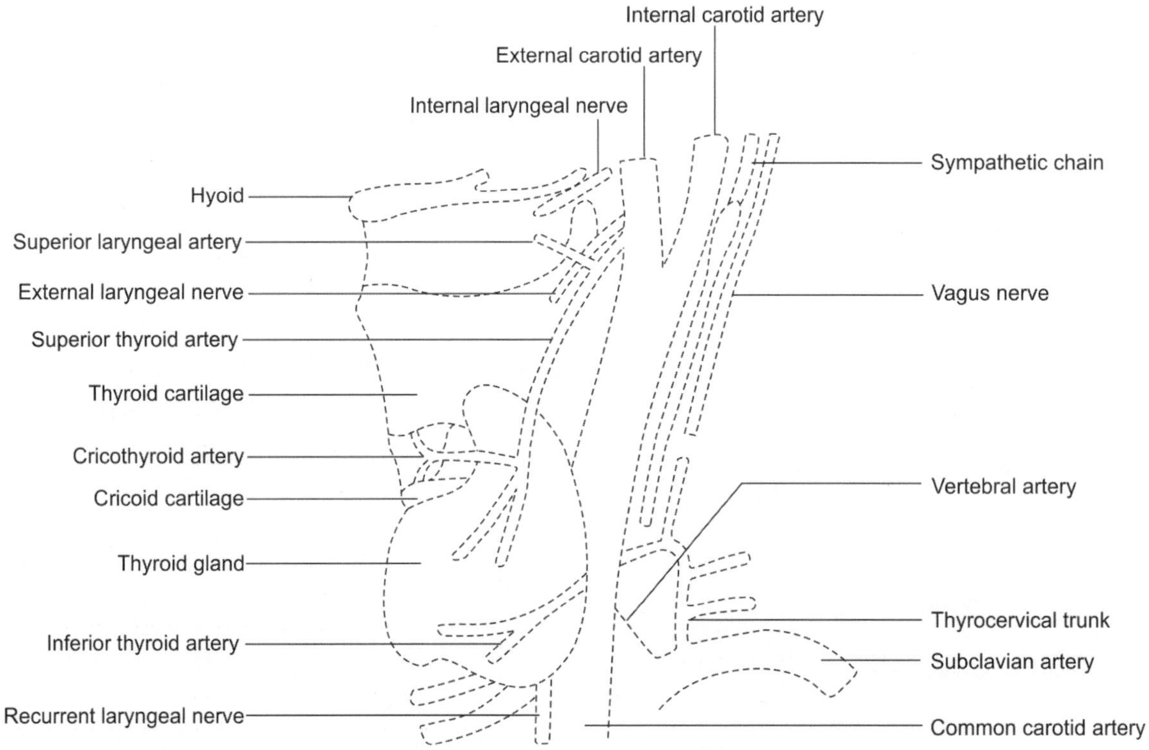

Figure 3.9: Thyroid gland—lateral view

KEY FEATURES

- It lies in front and side of neck opposite $C_{5\text{-}7}$, T_1
- It has two lobes which extend from oblique line of thyroid cartilage to 5-6 tracheal rings
- Two lobes are united by an isthmus which lies opposite to 2–4 tracheal rings
- It has a false capsule derived from pretracheal fascia which thickens to form suspensory ligament of Berry which connects it to cricoid. Thus, swellings of thyroid move with deglutition
- It is supplied by superior thyroid artery (branch of external carotid artery) which is accompanied by external laryngeal nerve and by inferior thyroid artery (branch of thyrocervical trunk) which is accompanied by recurrent laryngeal nerve.

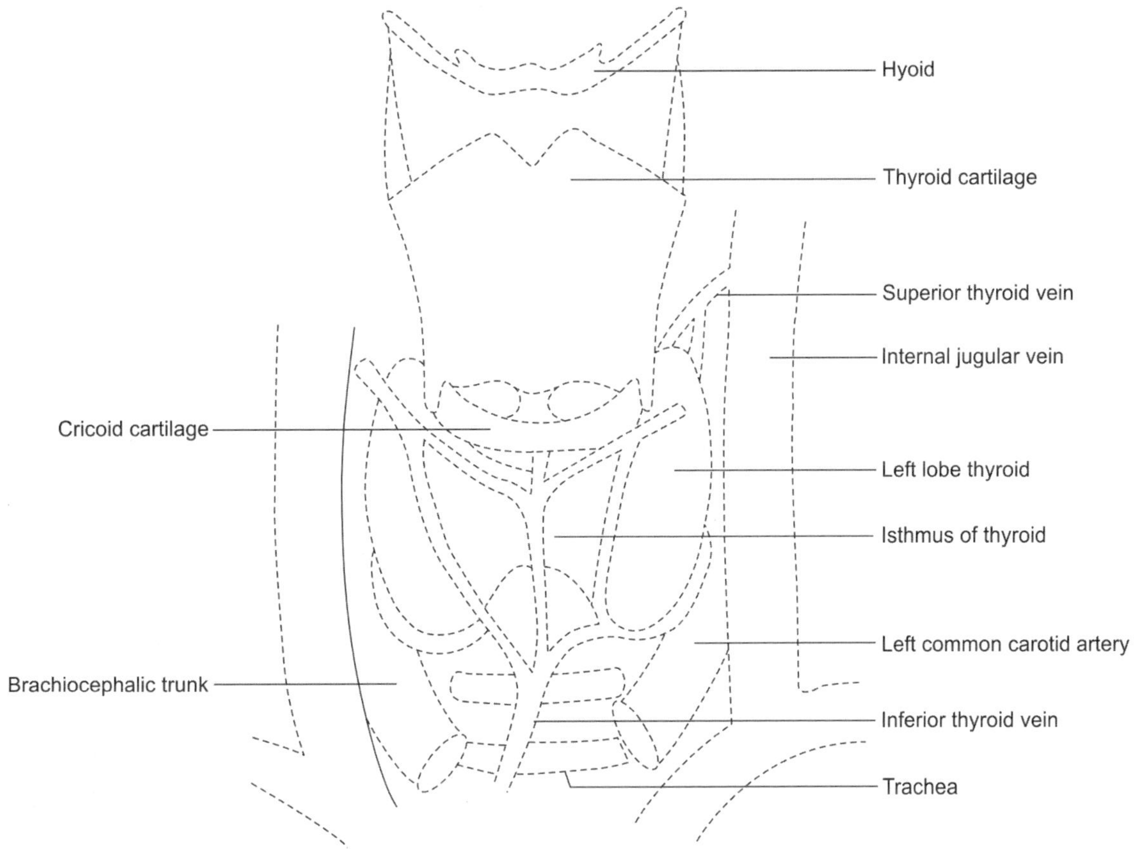

Figure 3.10: Thyroid gland—anterior view

KEY FEATURES

- The thyroid gland is drained by following veins:
  - Superior
  - Middle—both drains into internal jugular vein
  - Inferior—drains into left brachiocephalic vein.
- During thyroidectomy superior thyroid artery is ligated close to apex so that external laryngeal nerve is not damaged. The inferior thyroid artery is ligated away from the base of thyroid so that recurrent laryngeal nerve is not damaged.

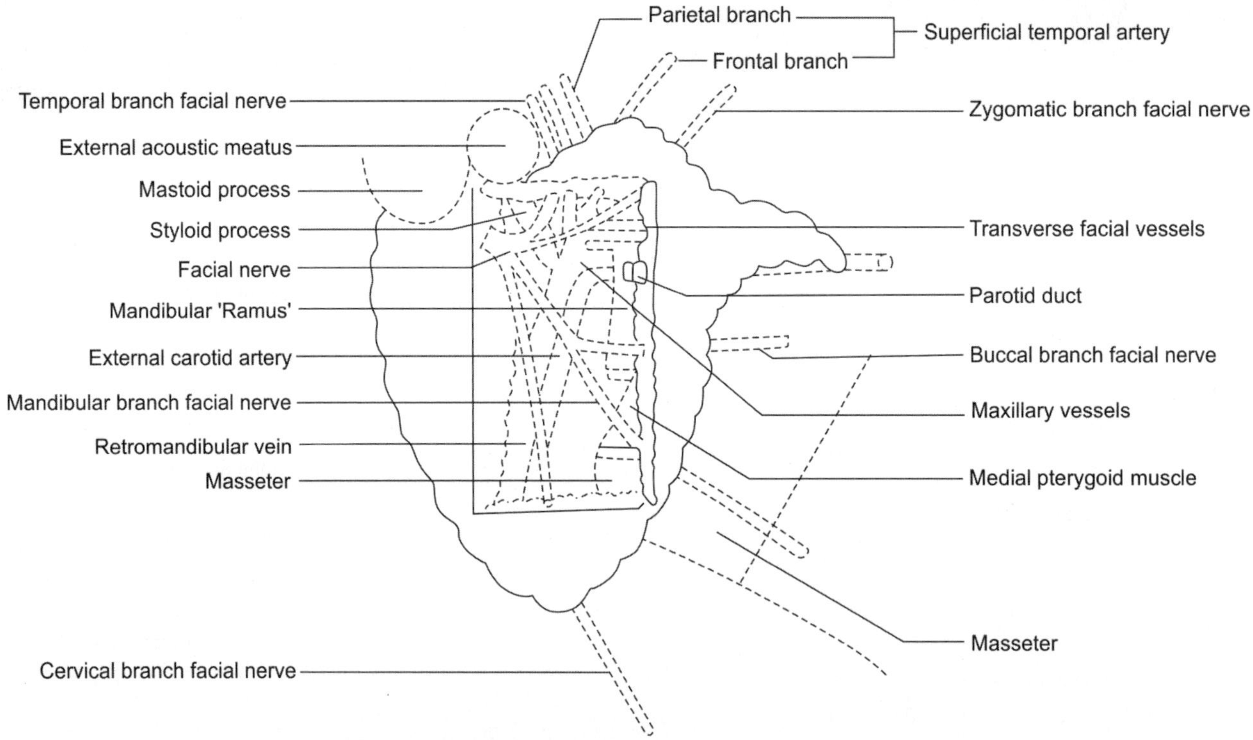

Figure 3.11: Parotid gland—window dissection

KEY FEATURES

- Its capsule is derived from deep cervical fascia hence swellings of parotid are painful
- Anteriorly related to—posterior border ramus of mandible, masseter and medial pterygoid muscles
- Posteriorly related to—mastoid process, posterior belly of digastric and stylohyoid muscles
- Superiorly related to—external acoustic meatus and posterior part of temporomandibular joint
- Medially related to—styloid process with three muscles, namely styloglossus, stylopharyngeus, stylohyoid along with two ligaments, namely stylomandibular and stylohyoid
- Structures passing through parotid:
  - Facial nerve and branches
  - Retromandibular vein
  - Terminal part of external carotid artery and its branches, namely posterior auricular, maxillary, superficial temporal and transverse facial.
- Injury to facial nerve during surgery can cause facial paralysis.

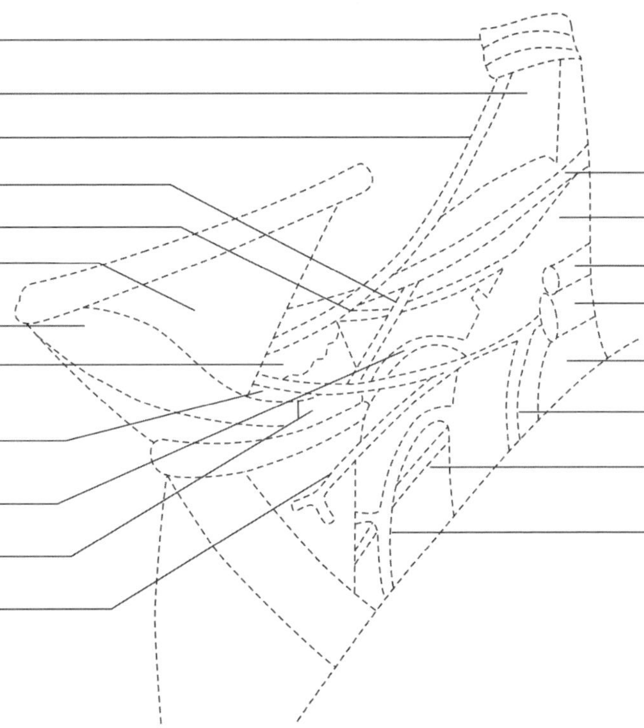

Figure 3.12: Submandibular region

KEY FEATURES

- Bounded by lower border mandible and two bellies of digastric muscle
- It contains suprahyoid muscles—digastric, stylohyoid, mylohyoid and geniohyoid
- Extrinsic muscles of tongue—hyoglossus, styloglossus and genioglossus
- It contains two glands, two arteries and two nerves:
  - Glands—submandibular and sublingual.
  - Arteries—lingual and facial.
  - Nerves—lingual and hypoglossal.
- The submandibular gland is enclosed by investing layer of deep fascia. It has two parts—superficial and deep with mylohyoid in between. The deep part lies between mylohyoid and hyoglossus.

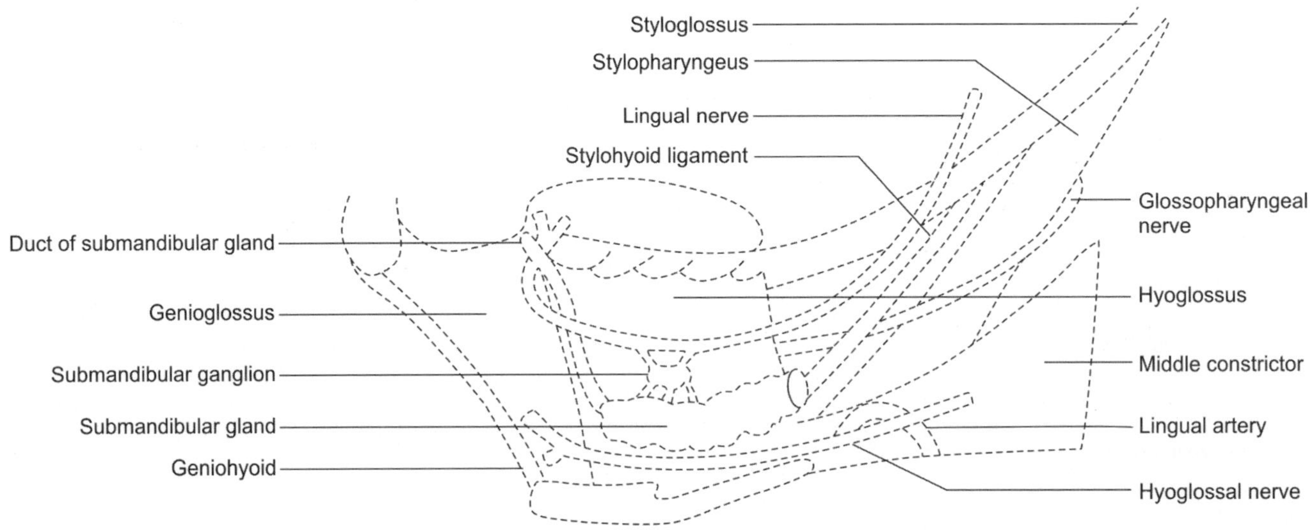

Figure 3.13: Superficial relations—hyoglossus

KEY FEATURES

- Deepest layer is formed by—geniohyoid, genioglossus and hyoglossus
- Structures superficial to hyoglossus are—hypoglossal nerve, lingual nerve, submandibular ganglion, deep part submandibular gland, styloglossus and mylohyoid
- Structures deep to hyoglossus—genioglossus anteriorly, middle constrictor posteriorly, inferior longitudinal muscle of tongue, 9th nerve, stylohyoid ligament and lingual artery.

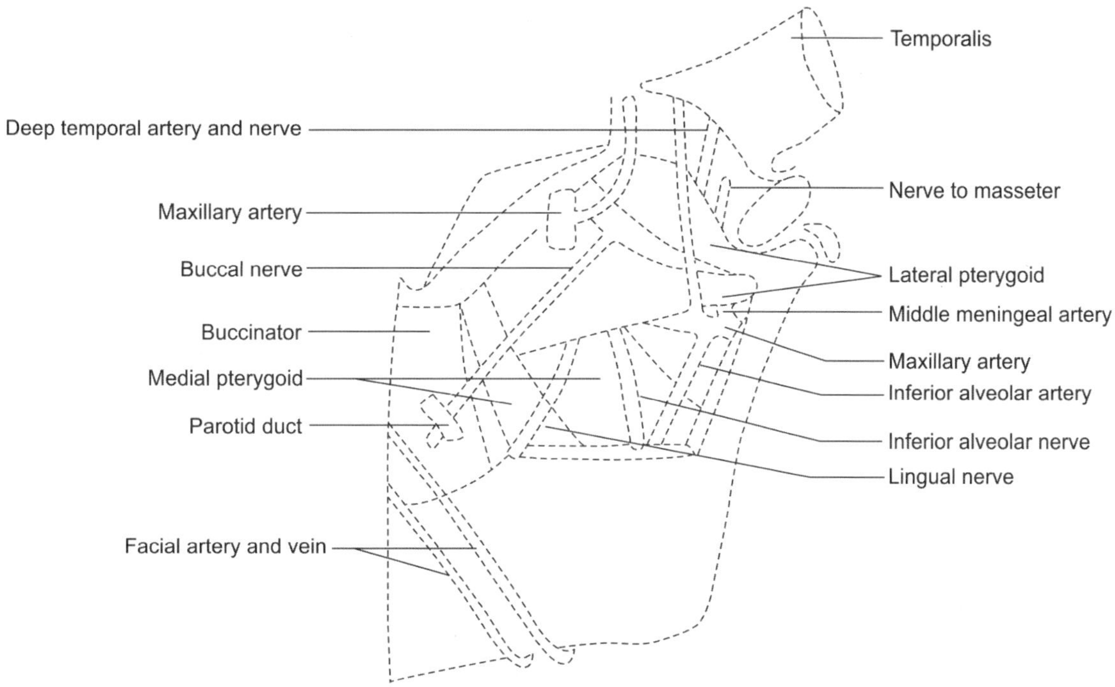

Figure 3.14: Infratemporal fossa

KEY FEATURES

- It is an area lying between lateral pterygoid plate medially and ramus of mandible laterally
- Maxilla anteriorly and styloid process posteriorly
- Contents:
  - Muscles—medial and lateral pterygoid, temporalis.
  - Vessels—maxillary artery, vein and pterygoid venous plexus.
  - Nerves—mandibular, chorda tympani and otic ganglion. Lateral pterygoid divides maxillary artery into three parts. Branches of 1st and 2nd part accompany branches of mandibular nerve whereas those of 3rd part accompany branches of maxillary nerve.

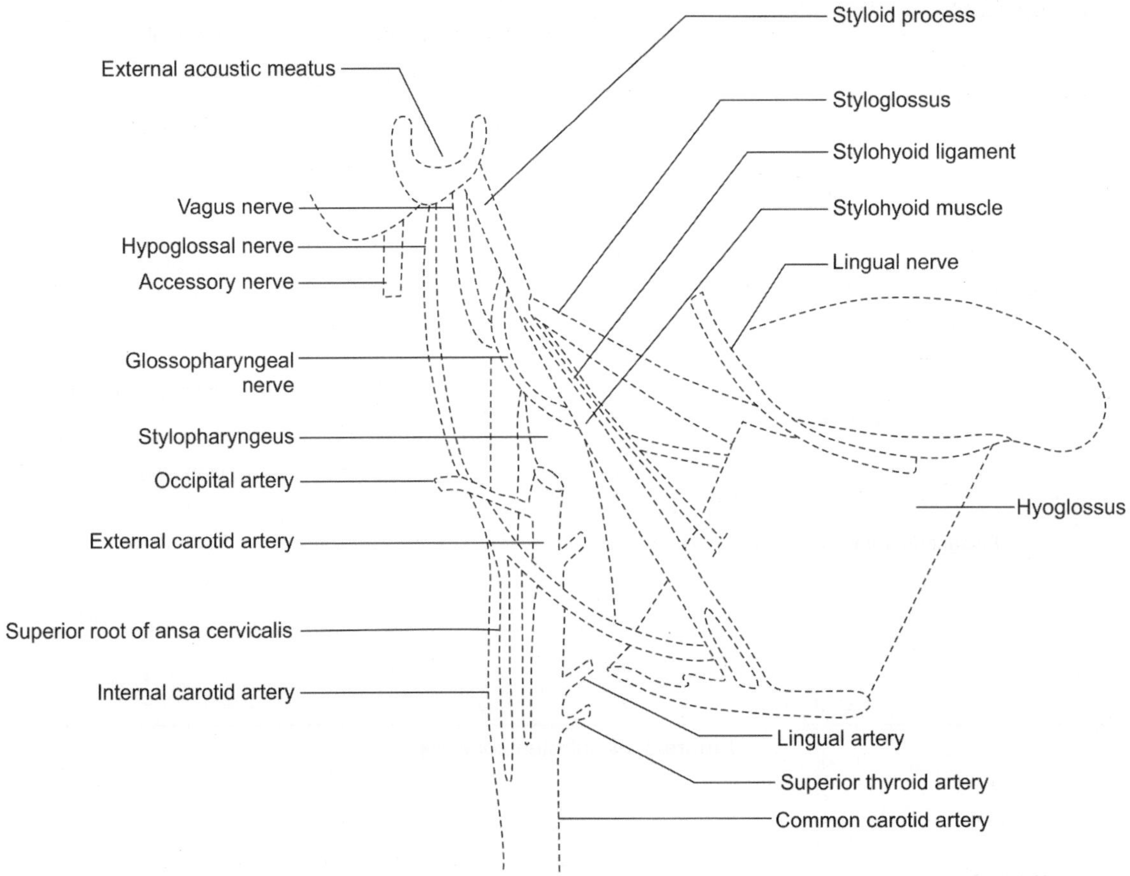

Figure 3.15: Styloid apparatus

KEY FEATURES

- It lies medial to parotid gland
- Styloid process gives attachment to three muscles and two ligaments:
  - Muscles:
    - Styloglossus supplied by hypoglossal nerve
    - Stylohyoid supplied by facial nerve
    - Stylopharyngeus supplied by glossopharyngeal nerve.
  - Ligaments:
    - Stylohyoid, a derivative of 2nd pharyngeal arch
    - Stylomandibular, a thickening of general investing fascia.

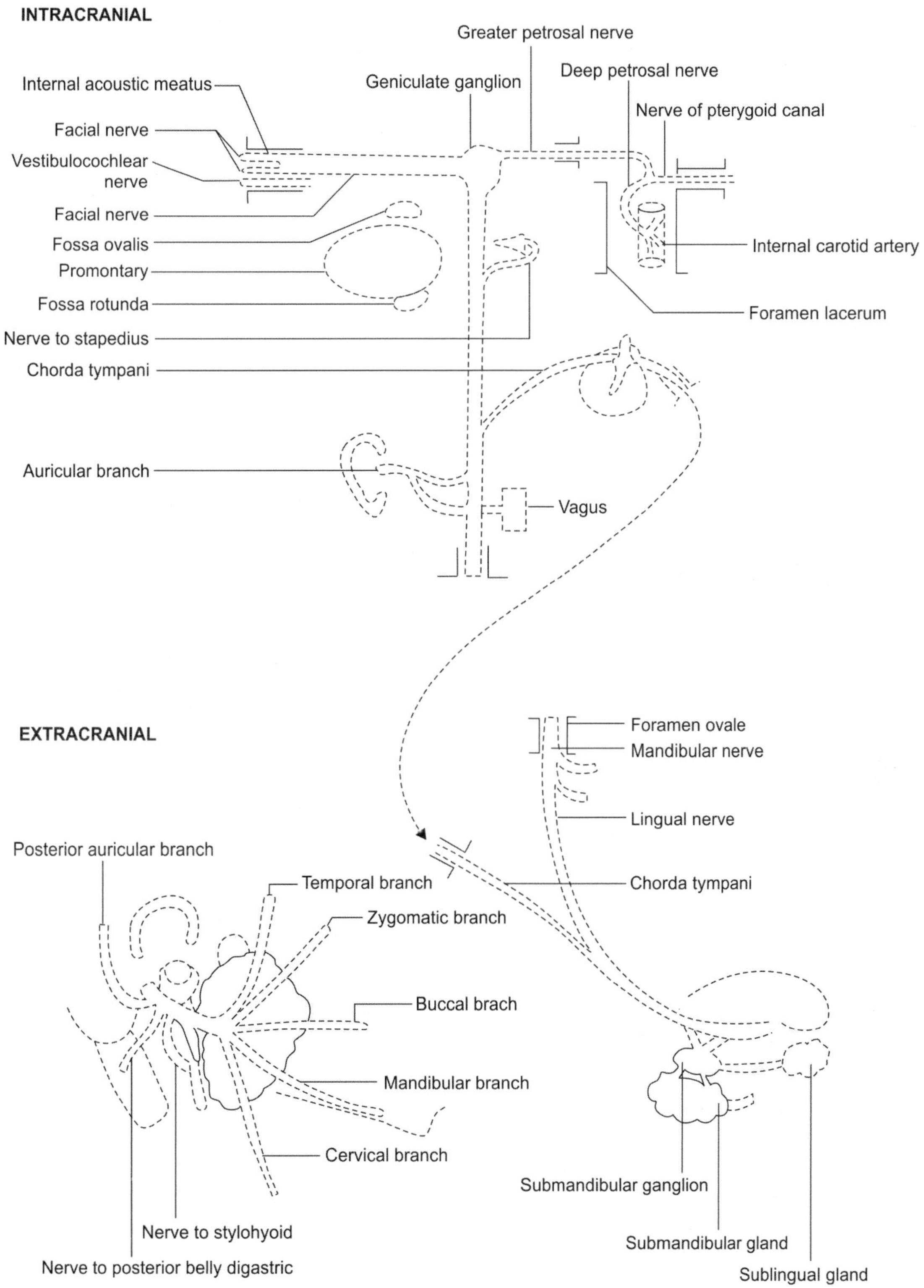

Figure 3.16: Facial nerve course—intracranial and extracranial

KEY FEATURES

- Mixed nerve but mainly motor
- Two motor nuclei:
  i. Motor nucleus supplies muscles of facial expression.
  ii. Superior salivatory and lacrimatory nucleus supplies submandibular, sublingual and lacrimal glands.
- Two sensory nuclei:
  i. Spinal nucleus of trigeminal receives general sensation from skin of auricle
  ii. Nucleus of tractus solitarius receives taste from anterior 2/3rd of tongue.
- Two roots:
  i. Large medial motor.
  ii. Small lateral sensory (nervus intermedius).
- Both the roots of facial nerve along with 8th nerve enter internal acoustic meatus
- Two roots of 7th nerve unite and enter facial canal in the medial wall of middle ear
- It bends at the junction of medial and posterior walls of middle ear to form geniculate ganglion
- It descends to emerge from stylomastoid foramen and curves forward to enter face by passing through parotid gland
- Lesions:
  - Supranuclear (upper motor neuron)—hemiplegia of lower half of face on opposite side only because upper half of the face has bilateral supply. In this case the lesion lies between cerebral cortex and the facial nucleus.
  - Infranuclear (lower motor neuron)—involves whole of the face on same side.
- The site of the lesion varies:
  - At geniculate ganglion—Bell's palsy, decreased salivation, loss of taste in anterior 2/3rd of tongue, hyperacusis (paralysis of stapedius) and loss of lacrimation.
  - Above the origin of nerve to stapedius—all signs and symptoms as in (a) but lacrimation is intact.
  - Above the origin of chorda tympani—Bell's palsy, decreased salivation, loss of taste in anterior 2/3rd of tongue.
  - At stylomastoid foramen—Bell's palsy—paralysis of muscles of facial expression. Mouth deviates to normal side, inability to close mouth and eye. Flattening of expression lines.

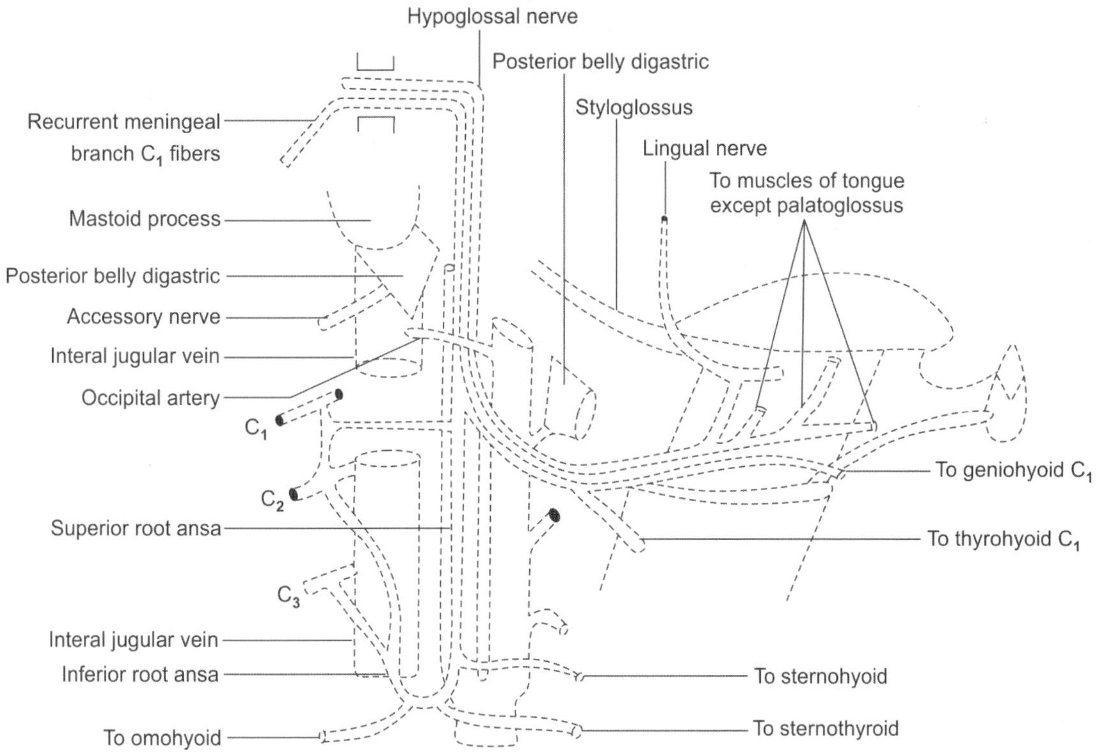

Figure 3.17: Hypoglossal nerve

KEY FEATURES

- Motor in nature and supplies all muscles of tongue except palatoglossus
- Its nucleus lies in the floor of 4th ventricle and emerges from medulla
- It comes out of the skull through hypoglossal canal
- It descends vertically downward and then curves forward in front of carotid arteries and lingual artery loop
- As it curves forward it is joined by fibers of C_1
- Some of the C_1 fibers leave hypoglossal nerve and descend as superior root of ansa cervicalis
- Rest of the fibers continue to supply geniohyoid and thyrohyoid muscles.

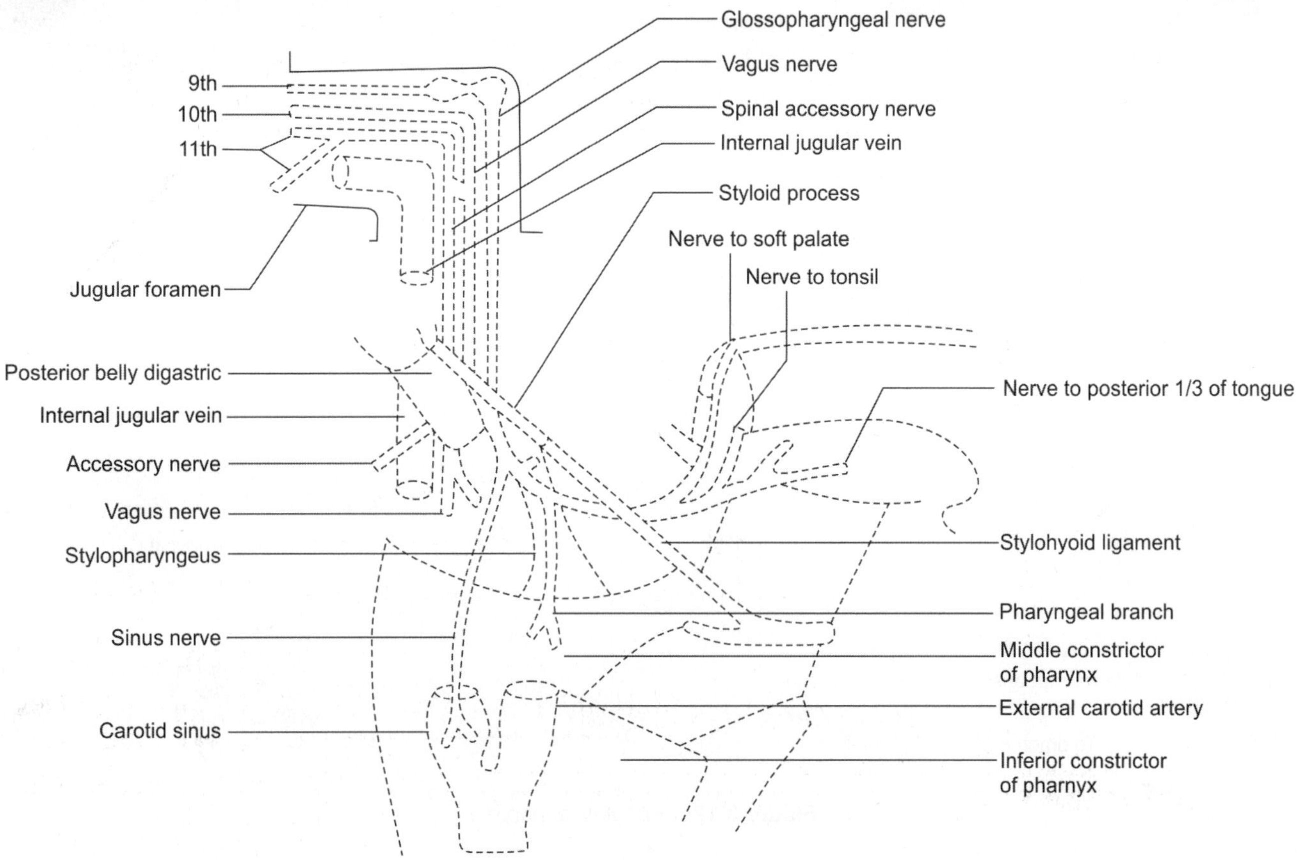

Figure 3.18: Glossopharyngeal nerve

KEY FEATURES

- It is a mixed nerve
- Motor nucleus:
  - Nucleus ambiguous supplies stylopharyngeus.
  - Inferior salivatory nucleus supplies secretomotor fibers to parotid.
- Sensory nucleus:
  - Nucleus of tractus solitarius receives taste from posterior 1/3rd of tongue.
  - Dorsal nucleus of vagus receives general sensations from pharynx, tonsil, soft palate and posterior 1/3rd of tongue.
  - Spinal nucleus of trigeminal receives proprioception from stylopharyngeus and skin of the auricle.
- Arises from medulla and leaves the skull through jugular foramen in a separate dural sheath along with 10th and 11th nerves
- It has superior and inferior sensory ganglia
- It runs down to reach styloid process, then follows stylopharyngeus through the gap between superior and middle constrictor of pharynx
- Then, turns forward to supply motor and sensory branches.

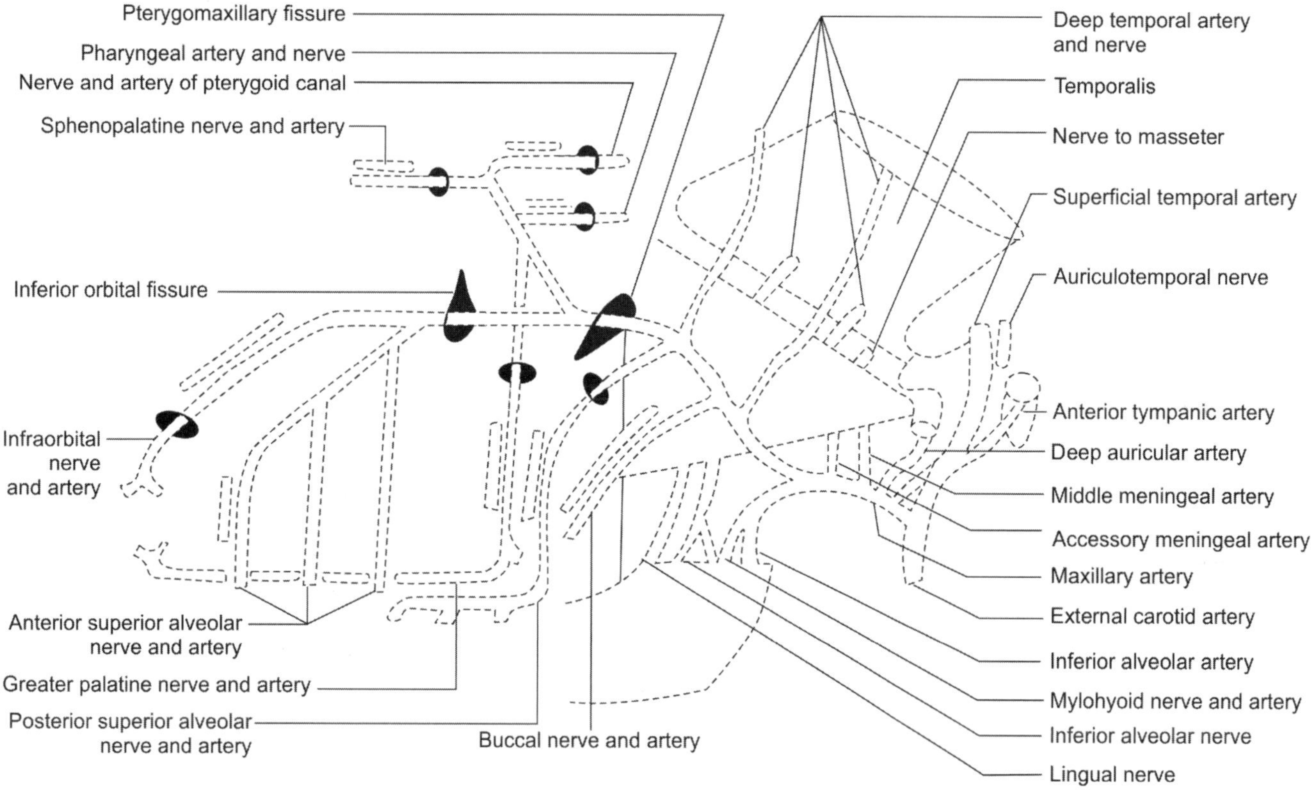

Figure 3.19: Maxillary artery

KEY FEATURES

- One of the terminal branches of external carotid artery
- Arises between neck of the mandible and sphenomandibular ligament
- Traverses infratemporal fossa, pterygopalatine fossa, floor of the orbit and continues on face as infraorbital artery
- It is divided into three parts by lower head lateral pterygoid into:
  i. mandibular
  ii. pterygoid
  iii. pterygopalatine.
- Branches of 1st and 2nd part accompany branches of mandibular nerve whereas branches of 3rd part accompany branches of maxillary nerve and pterygopalatine ganglion
- Most of the branches of maxillary artery pass through foramina and fissures.

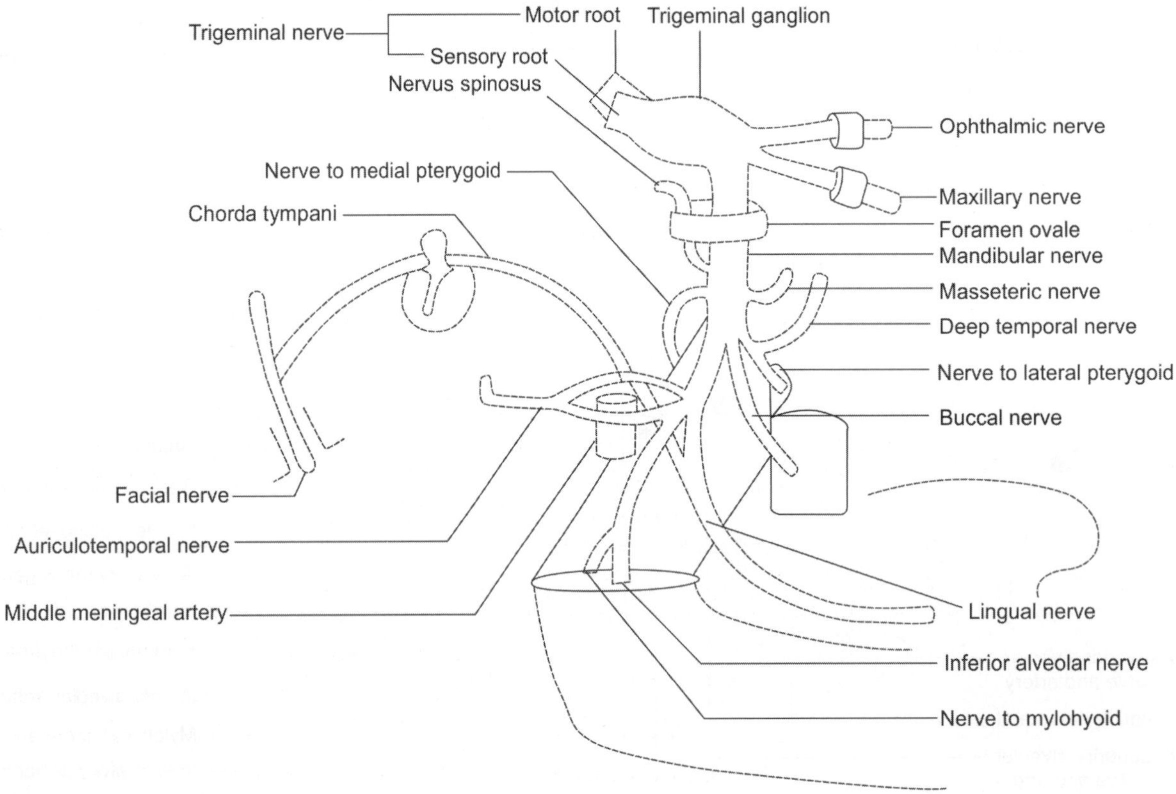

Figure 3.20: Mandibular nerve

KEY FEATURES

- Largest of the three divisions of trigeminal nerve
- Has a large sensory and small motor root
- Motor root arises from pons and in middle cranial fossa lies deep to trigeminal ganglion
- Sensory root arises from trigeminal ganglion
- Both the roots leave skull through foramen ovale and unite to form a single trunk to enter infratemporal fossa
- Below foramen ovale mandibular nerve divides into small anterior and large posterior branch
- All branches of anterior division are motor except buccal nerve which supplies mucous membrane of gums and cheeks
- All branches of posterior division are sensory except nerve to mylohyoid.

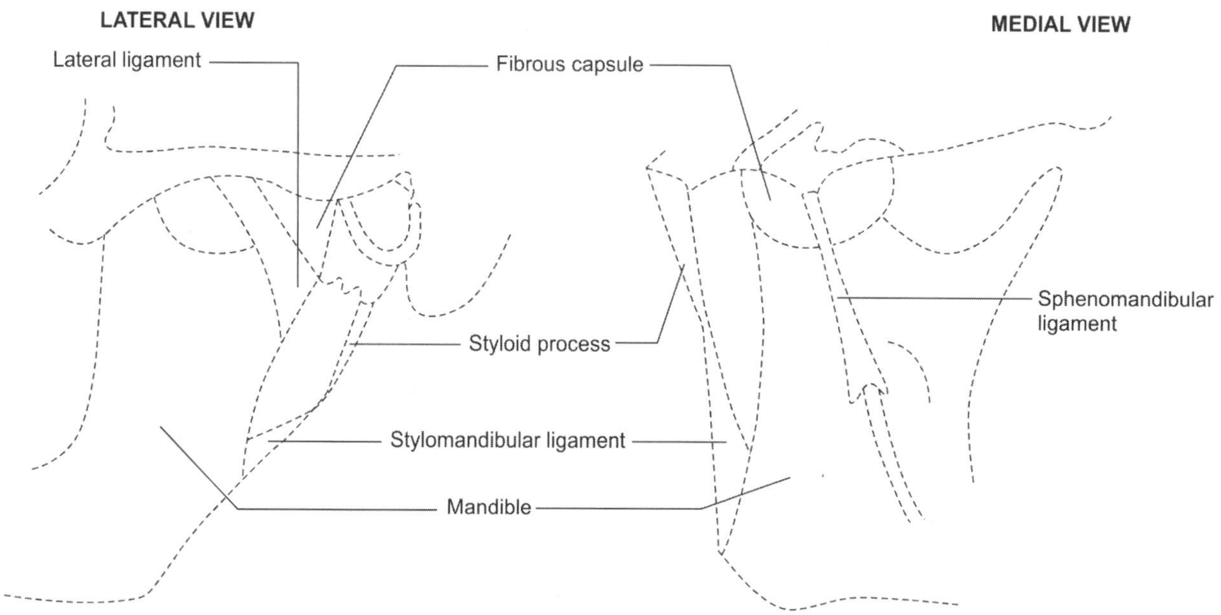

Figure 3.21: Temporomandibular joint

KEY FEATURES

- Atypical synovial joint with articular surfaces covered by fibrocartilage
- It is formed between head of the mandible and base of the skull
- The joint cavity is divided into upper and lower cavities by an articular disc (fibrocartilage)
- In upper cavity only gliding whereas in lower cavity gliding and rotation takes place
- Ligaments:
  - Fibrous capsule: Loose above articular disc and tight below the disc
  - Lateral: (Temporomandibular ligament) It is a true ligament
  - Sphenomandibular: Not a true ligament but is a derivative of 1st pharyngeal arch
  - Stylomandibular: Not a true ligament but is a condensation of deep cervical fascia.

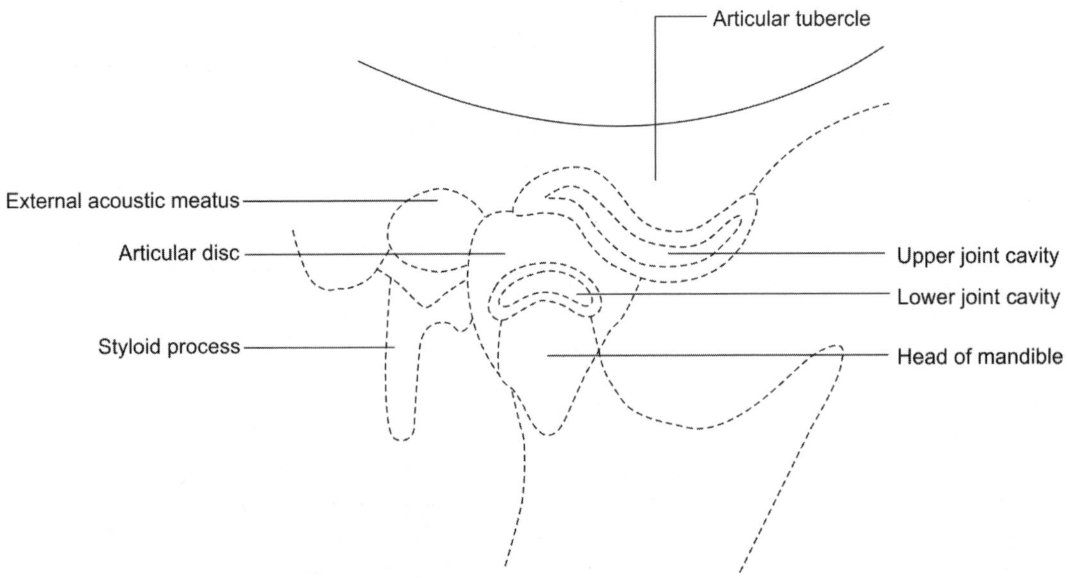

Figure 3.22: Temporomandibular joint—section

KEY FEATURES

- The articular surfaces of TM joint are not congruent hence the need for an articular disc
- Upper articular surface is concavo-convex whereas inferior surface is concave
- The disc is firmly attached to capsule
- Anteriorly extends through capsule and becomes continuous with the tendon of lateral pterygoid muscle
- In depression of mandible (opening of mouth) movement occurs in upper compartment, i.e. lateral pterygoid and head of the mandible move as a unit
- Right and left TM joints move together.

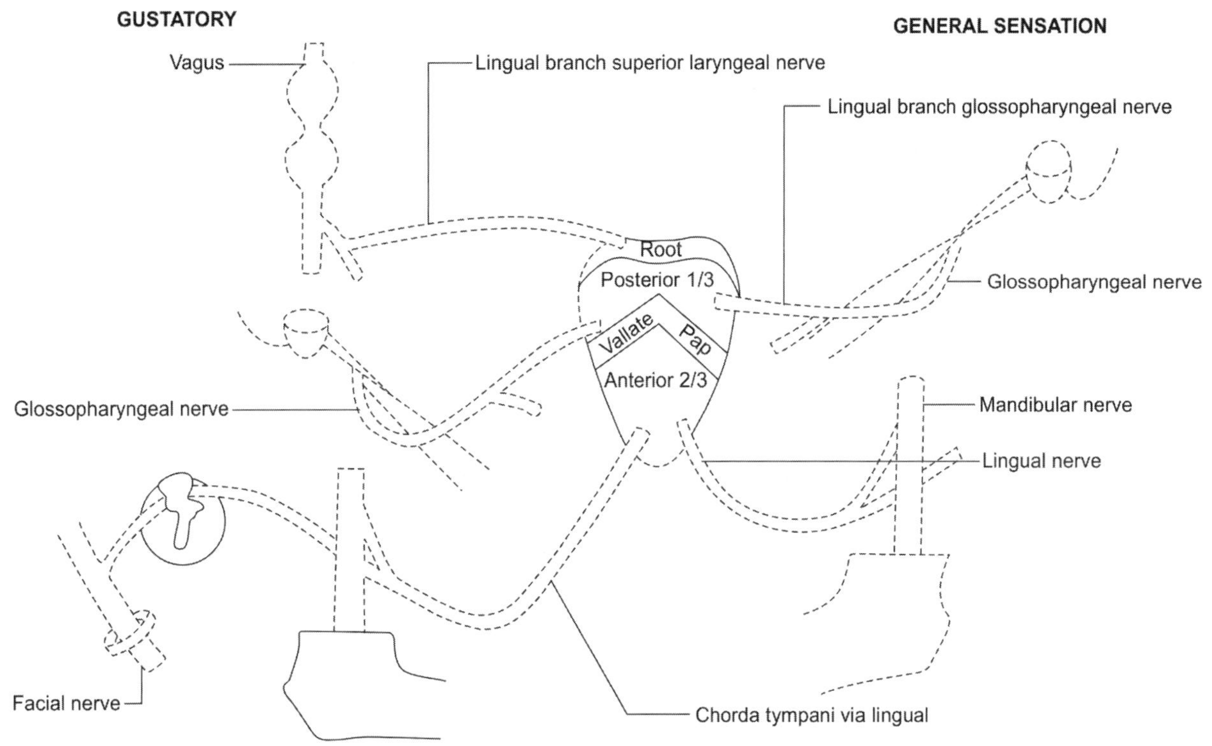

Figure 3.23: Nerve supply of tongue—gustatory and general sensation

KEY FEATURES

- Anterior 2/3rd of tongue:
  - Lingual nerve pretrematic nerve of 1st pharyngeal arch.
  - Gustatory (taste)—chorda tympani via lingual nerve.
  - General sensation—lingual nerve.
- Posterior 1/3rd of tongue: Glossopharyngeal nerve of 3rd arch carries both gustatory and general sensation
- Root of tongue: Superior laryngeal nerve of 4th pharyngeal arch carries both gustatory and general sensation.

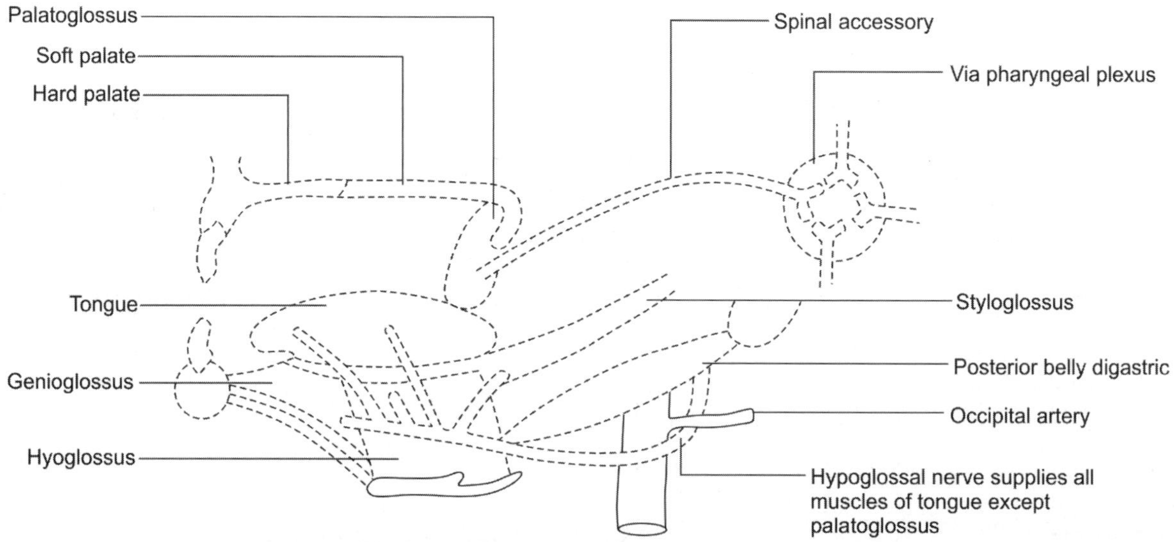

Figure 3.24: Motor nerve supply of tongue

KEY FEATURES

- All muscles of tongue are supplied by hypoglossal nerve except palatoglossus which is supplied by pharyngeal plexus
- Genioglossus—protrusion of tongue; styloglossus—retraction of tongue; hyoglossus—depression of tongue; palatoglossus—elevation of tongue. Intrinsic muscles—causes change in shape.

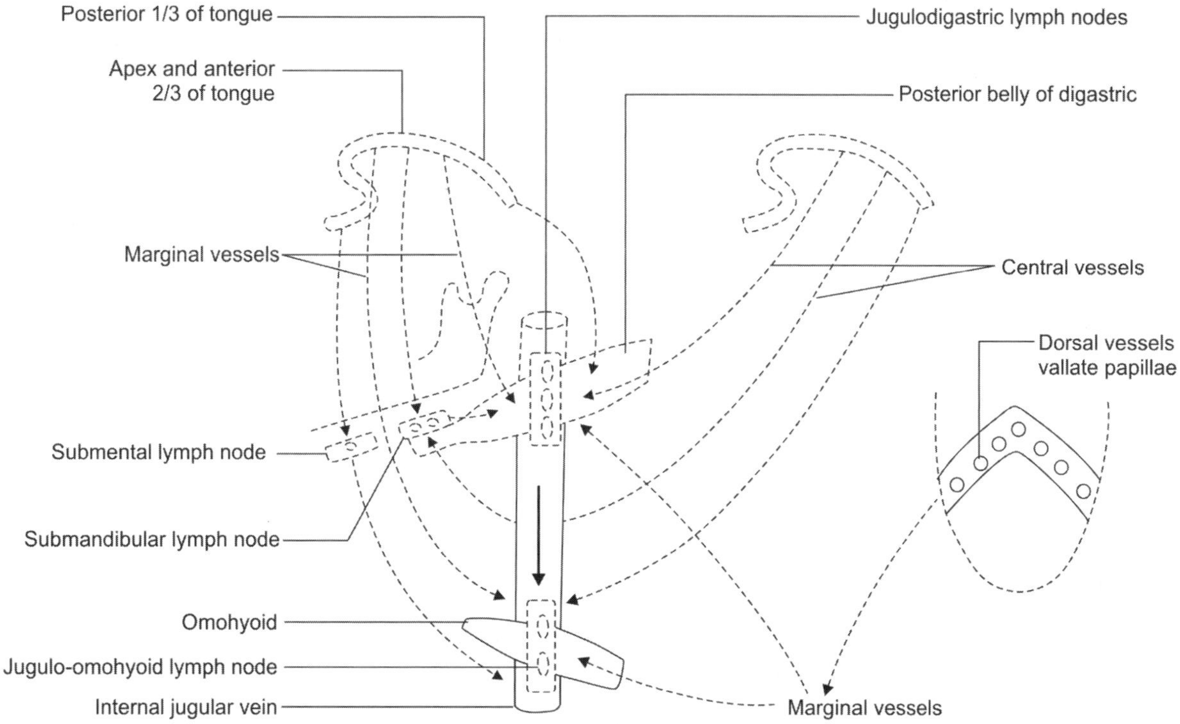

Figure 3.25: Lymphatic drainage of tongue

KEY FEATURES

- Apical region drains into submental to submandibular and some cross to reach jugulodigastric lymph nodes
- Anterior 2/3rd marginal area drains into submandibular to lower deep cervical lymph nodes
- Anterior 2/3rd central area drains into deep cervical lymph nodes
- Posterior 1/3rd basal area drains bilaterally into deep cervical and jugulodigastric lymph nodes
- Lymphatics of posterior 1/3rd right and left side, freely communicate with each other hence metastasis of carcinoma tongue has poor prognosis.

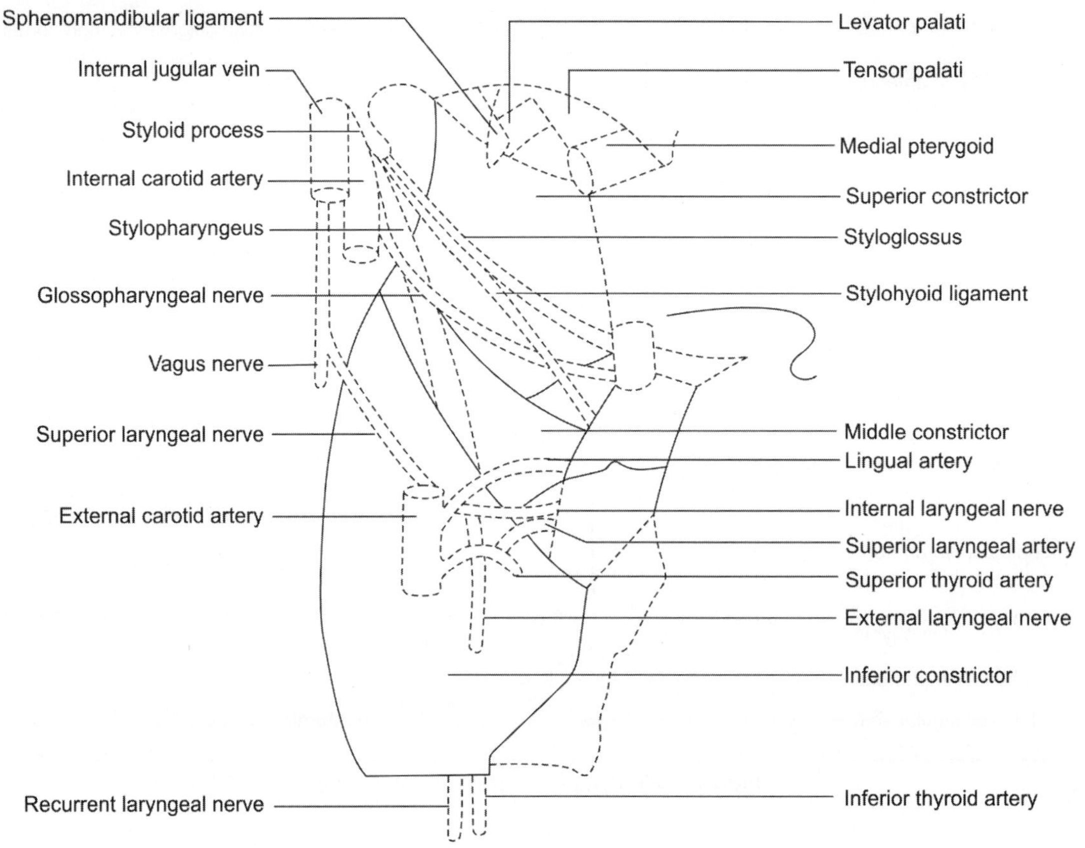

Figure 3.26: Constrictors of pharynx—relations

KEY FEATURES

- Three in number, superior constrictor is innermost whereas inferior constrictor is outermost
- Collectively they form a muscular tube which is open anteriorly to communicate with nasal cavity, oral cavity and larynx
- Thus, pharynx is divided into nasopharynx, oropharynx and laryngopharynx
- Nasopharynx extends from base of skull to soft palate, has pharyngeal tonsil and opening of auditory tube
- Oropharynx extends from soft palate to upper border of epiglottis, has palatine tonsil
- Laryngopharynx extends from upper border of epiglottis to lower border of cricoid cartilage
- Between base of skull and upper free border of superior constrictor lies pharyngo-basilar fascia which is pierced by auditory tube, tensor palati and ascending pharyngeal artery
- Between superior and middle constrictor lies stylopharyngeus and glossopharyngeal nerve
- Between middle and inferior constrictor lies superior and internal laryngeal artery.

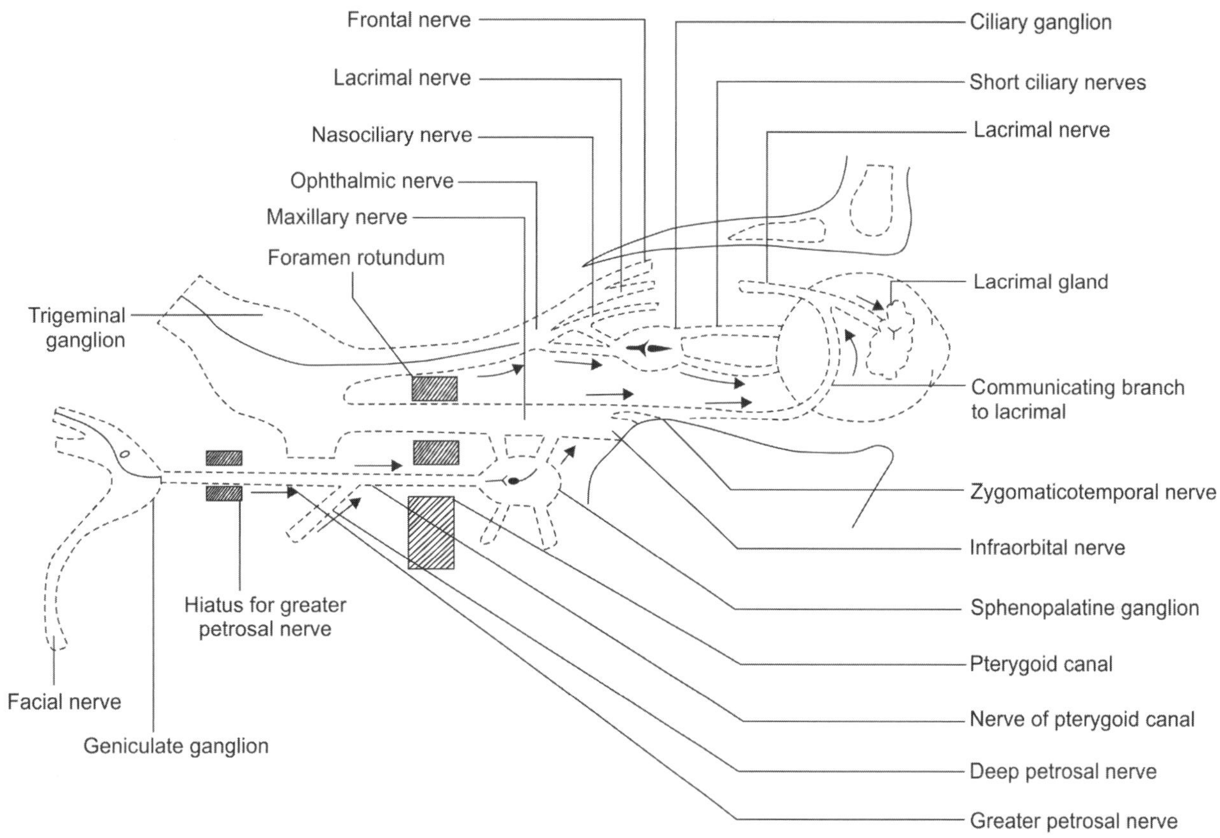

Figure 3.27: Parasympathetic ganglia—Ciliary and sphenopalatine

KEY FEATURES

- **Sphenopalatine ganglion***:* Largest topographically related to maxillary nerve but functionally related to facial nerve through greater petrosal nerve.
  - Motor root—fibers relay and supply secretomotor to lacrimal gland, mucous glands of nose, palate, pharynx and paranasal sinuses.
  - Sympathetic root—vasomotor fibers pass through the ganglion and supply lacrimal gland, mucous glands of nose, palate, pharynx and paranasal sinuses.
  - Sensory root—they are the branches of maxillary nerve.
- **Ciliary ganglion:** Topographically related to nasociliary nerve but functionally related to occulomotor nerve.
  - Motor root—fibers arise from Edinger-Westphal nucleus, relay in the ganglion and supply ciliary muscle and sphincter pupillae.
  - Sympathetic root—supplies dilator pupillae and blood vessels of eye ball.
  - Sensory root—they are the branches of nasociliary nerve and carry pain, touch and temperature from eye ball.

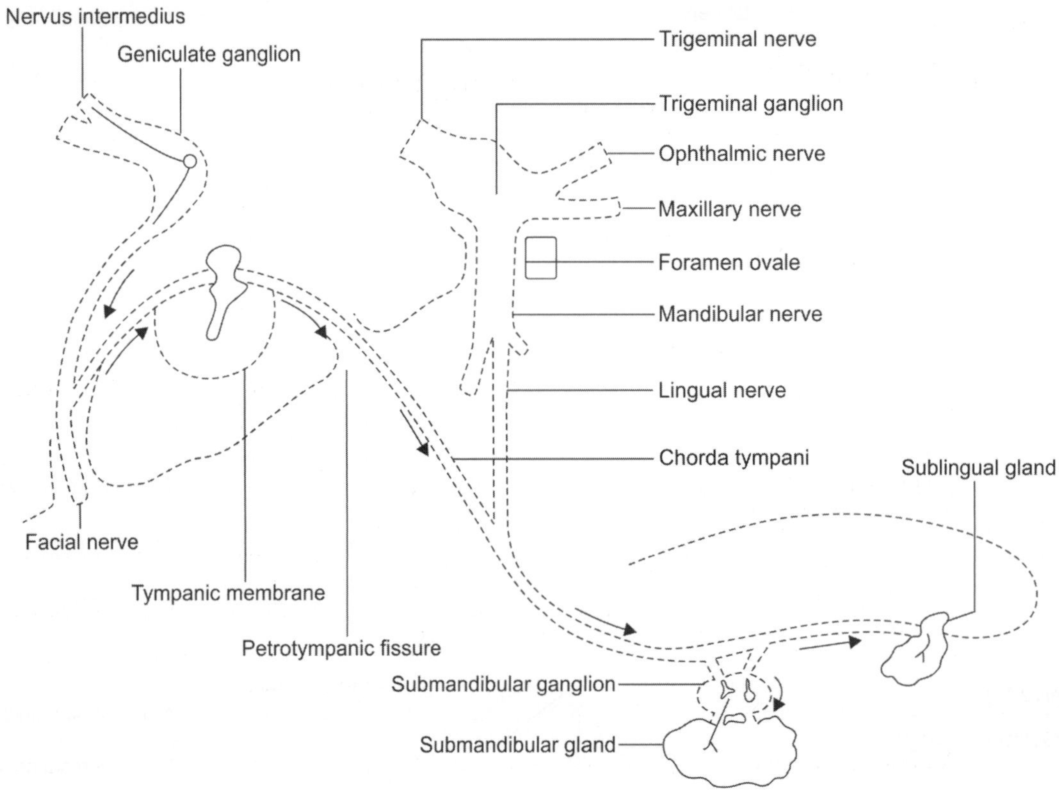

Figure 3.28: Submandibular ganglion

KEY FEATURES

- Topographically related to lingual nerve but functionally related to facial nerve through chorda tympani
- Motor root—fibers arise from superior salivatory nucleus, relay in the ganglion and supply submandibular and sublingual glands
- Sympathetic root—supplies vasomotor fibers to submandibular and sublingual glands
- Sensory root—arises from lingual nerve.

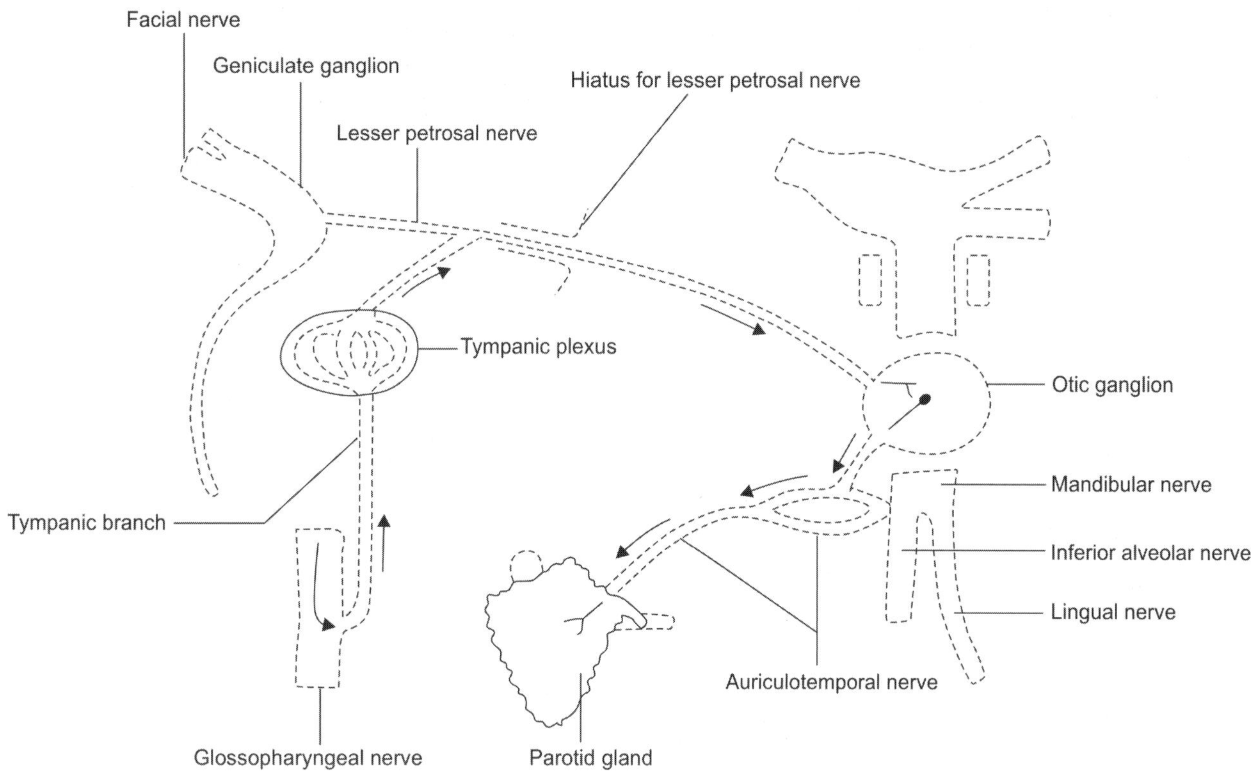

Figure 3.29: Otic ganglion

KEY FEATURES

- Topographically related to mandibular nerve but functionally related to glossopharyngeal nerve
- Motor root—supplies secretomotor fibers to parotid gland after relay in otic ganglion
- Sympathetic root—supplies vasomotor fibers to parotid gland via auriculotemporal nerve
- Sensory root—from auriculotemporal nerve
- Somatic motor—supplies medial pterygoid, tensor palati and tensor tympani.

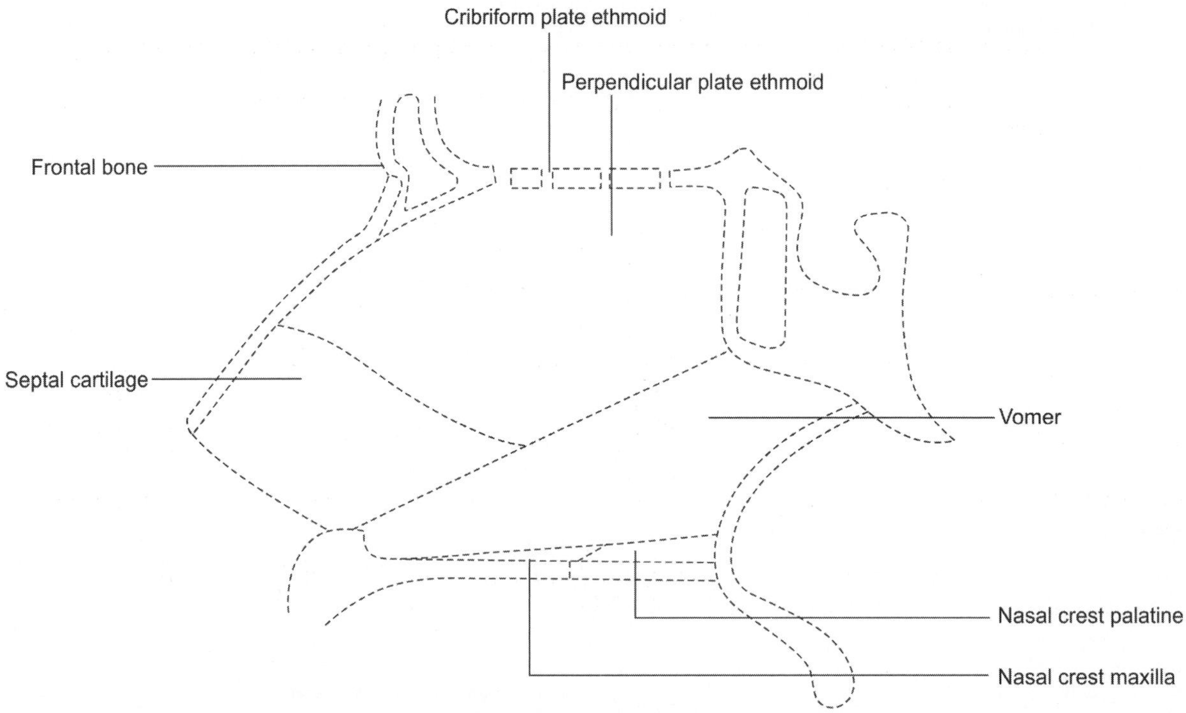

Figure 3.30: Nasal septum

KEY FEATURES

- It is an osteocartilagenous partition
- Bony part—perpendicular plate of ethmoid posterosuperiorly
  - Vomer forms posteroinferior part
  - Nasal spine frontal bone
  - Nasal crest of nasal bones, sphenoid and palatine process of maxilla
- Cartilagenous part—septal cartilage
  - Septal process of two major alar cartilages
- Membranous part—fibrous tissue with double layer of skin.

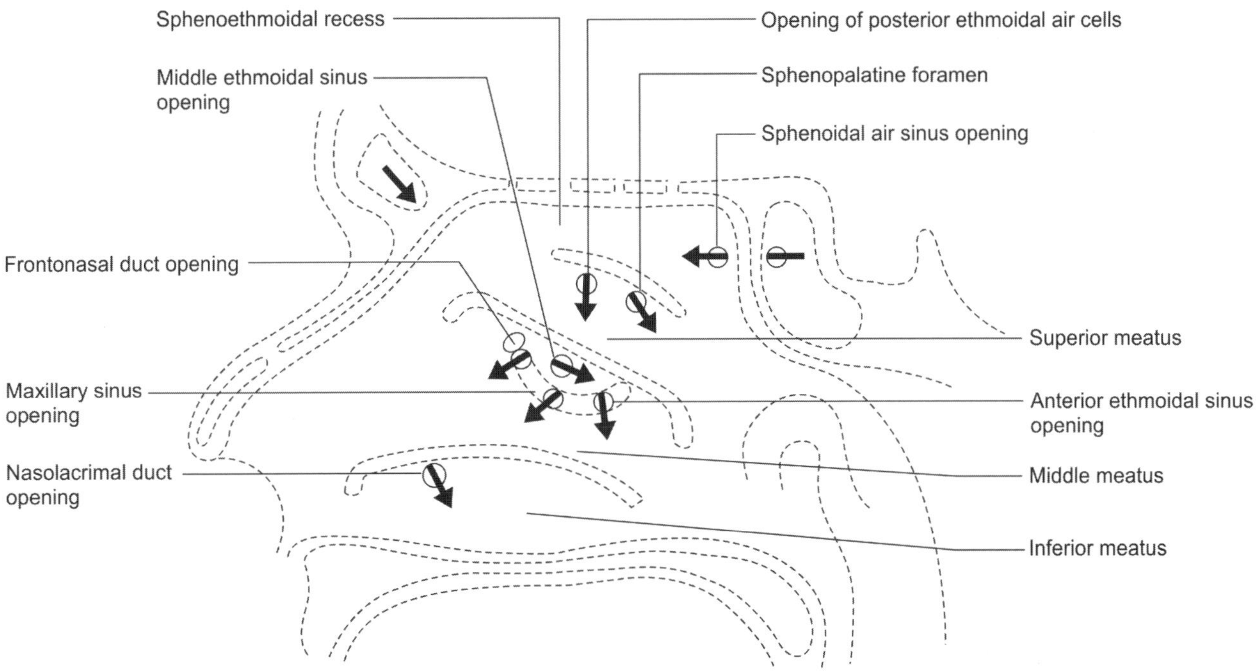

Figure 3.31: Lateral wall of nose

KEY FEATURES

- It shows three elevations called conchae which cover three meatuses
- Superior and middle conchae are parts of ethmoid bone
- Above the superior meatus there is sphenoethmoidal recess in which sphenoidal air sinus opens
- Superior meatus is smallest, posterior ethmoidal air cells and sphenopalatine foramen opens
- In middle meatus anterior and middle ethmoidal air cells, frontonasal duct and maxillary air sinus opens
- In inferior meatus nasolacrimal duct opens.

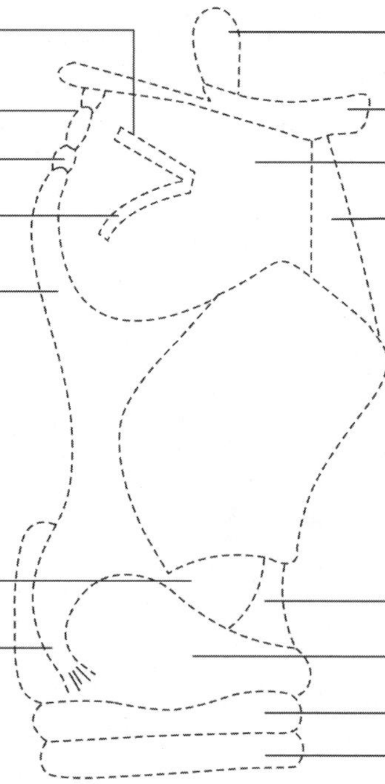

Figure 3.32: Larynx—lateral view

KEY FEATURES

- Larynx has three unpaired cartilages—thyroid, cricoid and epiglottis and three paired cartilages—arytenoid, corniculate and cuneiform
- Thyroid cartilage is attached above to hyoid by median and lateral thyrohyoid ligaments and thyrohyoid membrane. This membrane is pierced by internal laryngeal nerve and superior laryngeal artery
- Below, the thyroid cartilage is attached to cricoid by anterior cricothyroid ligament and cricovocal membrane
- Epiglottis is attached to thyroid cartilage by thyroepiglottic ligament and to hyoid by hyoepiglottic ligament.

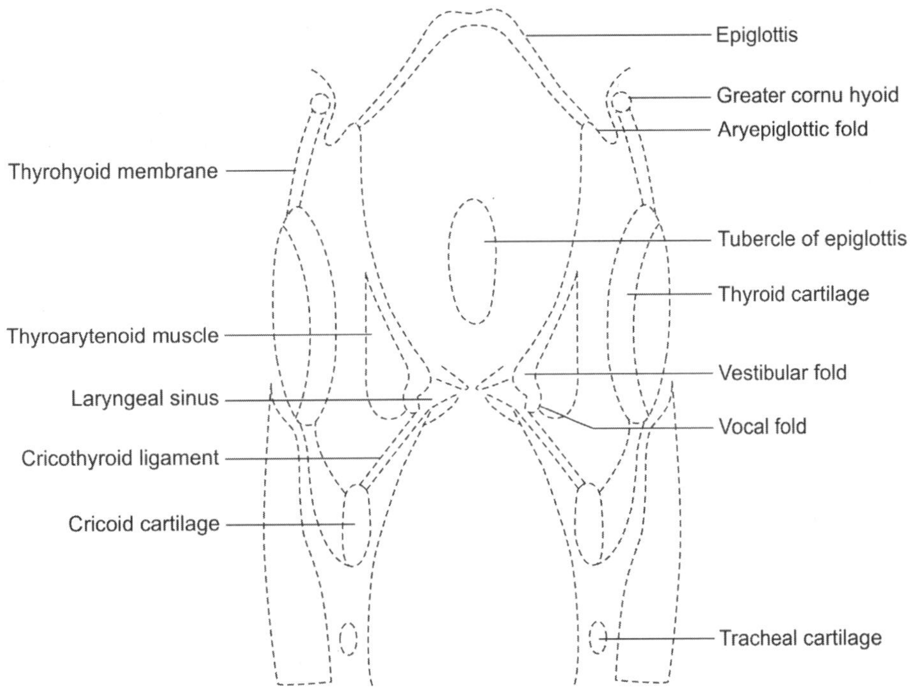

Figure 3.33: Larynx—coronal section

KEY FEATURES

- Larynx can be divided in three parts—supraglottic, glottic and infraglottic
  i. Supraglottic part (vestibule of larynx) extends from inlet of larynx to vestibular folds.
  ii. Glottic part also called ventricles or sinus of larynx) lies between vestibular and vocal folds. It is a diverticulum of mucous membrane.
  iii. Infraglottic part extends from vocal folds to lower border of cricoid cartilage.
- Arterial supply:
  - Above vocal fold supplied by superior laryngeal artery branch of superior thyroid artery.
  - Below vocal fold supplied by inferior laryngeal artery branch of inferior thyroid artery.
- Motor supply—intrinsic muscles of larynx are supplied by recurrent laryngeal nerve except cricothyroid which is supplied by external laryngeal nerve
- Posterior cricoarytenoids are the only abductor of vocal folds, hence safety muscle of larynx rest all intrinsic muscles are adductors of the vocal folds.

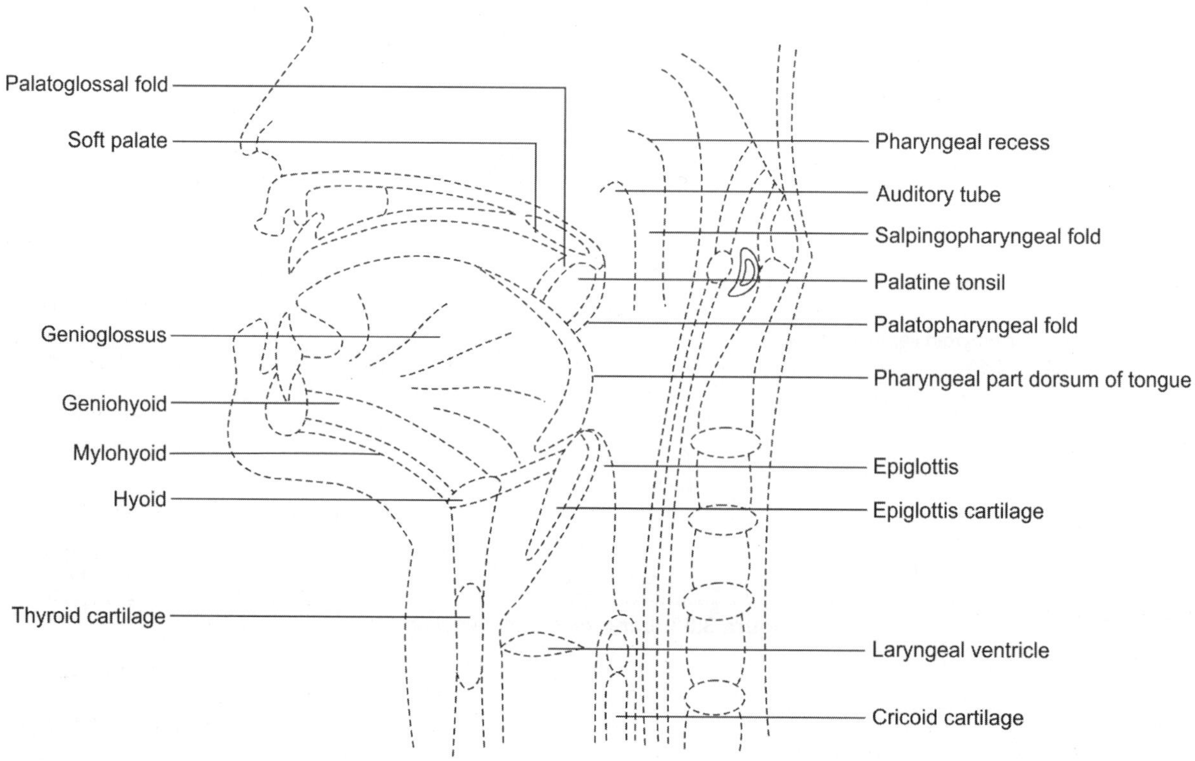

Figure 3.34: Paramedian section—head and neck

KEY FEATURES

- Showing oral cavity, larynx and pharynx
- In oral cavity, there are two palatine tonsils lying between palatoglossus and palatopharyngeal folds. Fibers of genioglossus are arranged in radiating pattern and form the safety muscle of the tongue
- The larynx extends from epiglottis to lower border of cricoid
- The pharynx communicates anteriorly with nasal cavity (nasopharynx), oral cavity (oropharynx) and larynx (laryngopharynx).

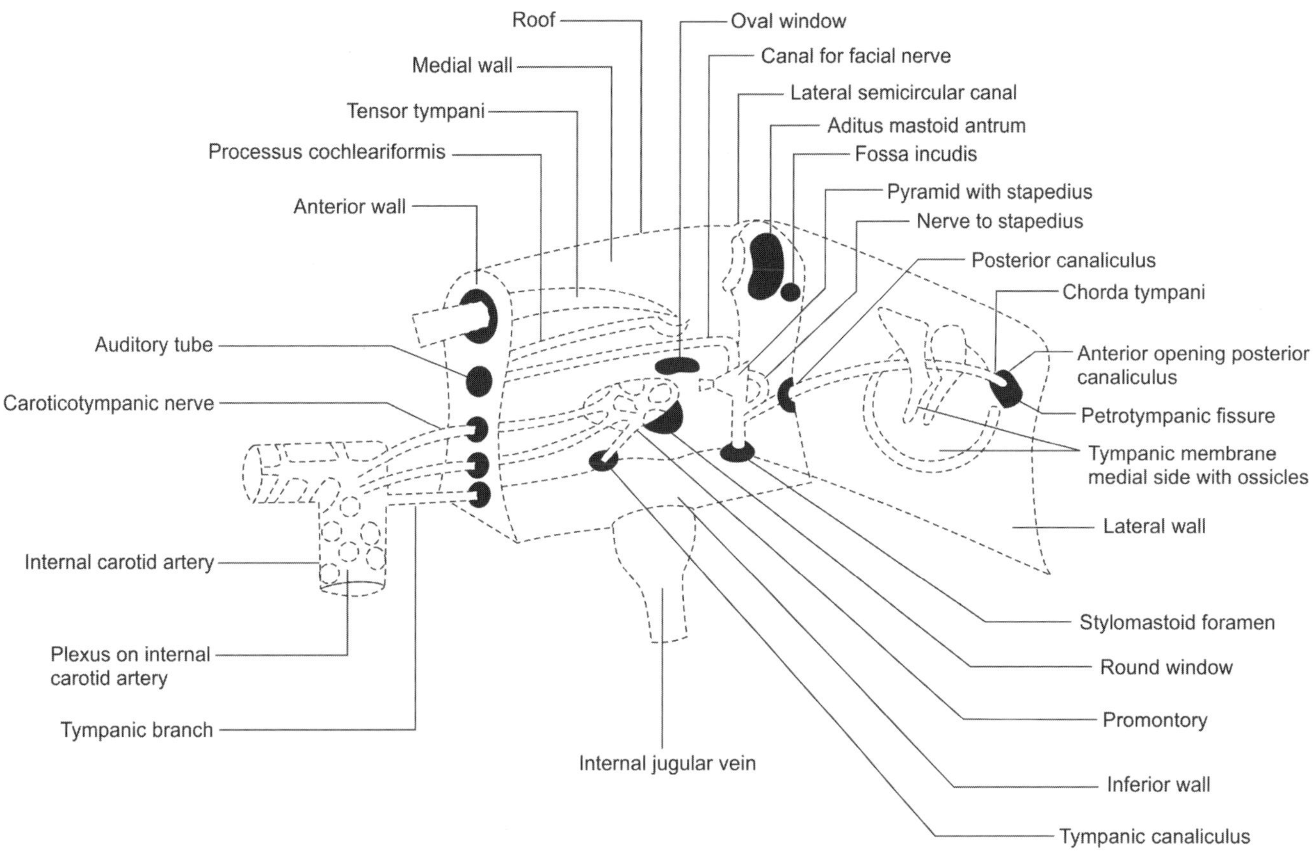

Figure 3.35: Middle ear cavity—lateral wall open

KEY FEATURES

- Located within petrous temporal bone and contains three ear ossicles—malleus, incus and stapes
- It has six walls:
  i. Lateral wall (tympanic wall) made up of tympanic membrane along with handle of malleus and chorda tympani nerve.
  ii. Medial wall (vestibular wall) made up of bony plate having promontory, oval window in which foot plate of stapes fits, round window, elevation raised by facial canal and processus trochleariformis over which tensor tympani changes direction.
  iii. Anterior wall (carotid wall) related to internal carotid artery. It has three openings for tensor tympani, auditory tube and caroticotympanic nerves.
  iv. Posterior wall (mastoid wall) related to mastoid antrum, fossa incudis, lateral semicircular canal and pyramid.
  v. Roof formed by tegmentum tympani.
  vi. Floor (jugular wall) related to bulb of internal jugular vein.
- The junction of medial and posterior wall is related to vertical part facial canal and stylomastoid foramen. At the junction of medial wall and floor there is tympanic canaliculus.

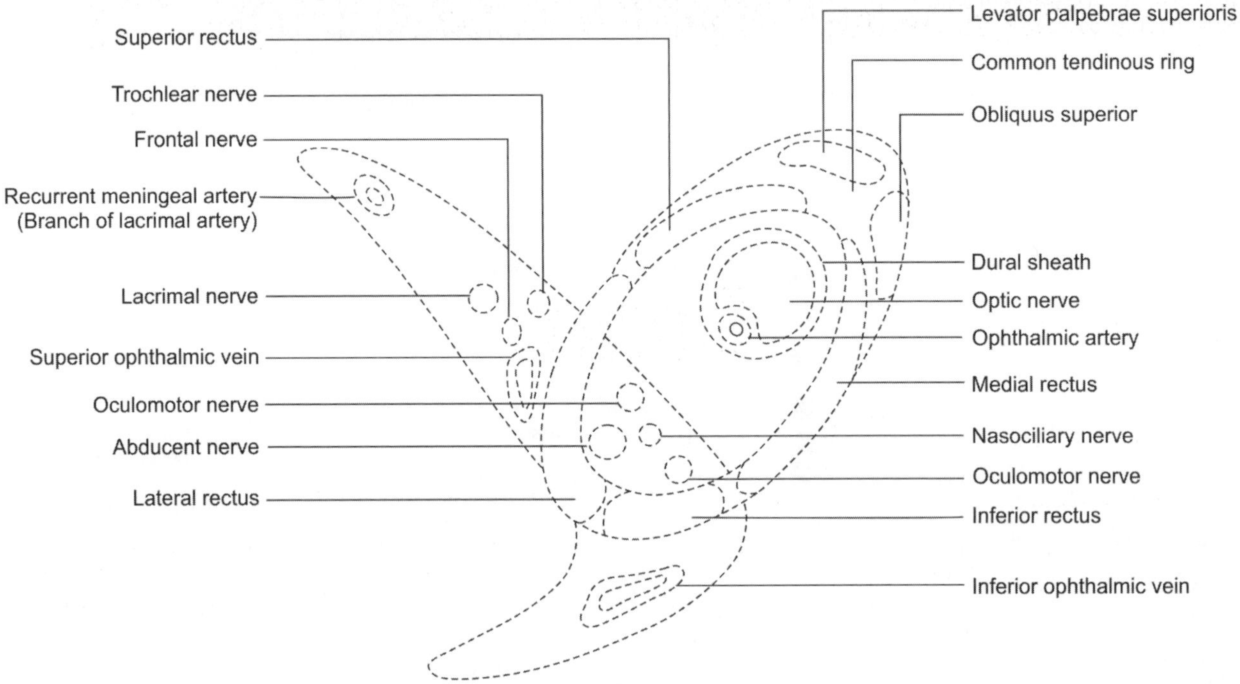

Figure 3.36: Superior orbital fissure

KEY FEATURES

- The bony orbit communicates with middle cranial fossa through superior orbital fissure
- The fissure is divided into three parts by a tendinous ring:
  i. Lateral part through which passes recurrent meningeal artery, lacrimal, frontal and trochlear nerves, superior ophthalmic vein.
  ii. Medial part through which passes inferior ophthalmic vein.
  iii. Middle part through which passes two divisions of occulomotor nerve, nasociliary nerve and abducent nerve.
- The tendinous ring gives attachment to extraocular muscles and also gives passage to optic nerve and ophthalmic artery.

CHAPTER 4

Brain

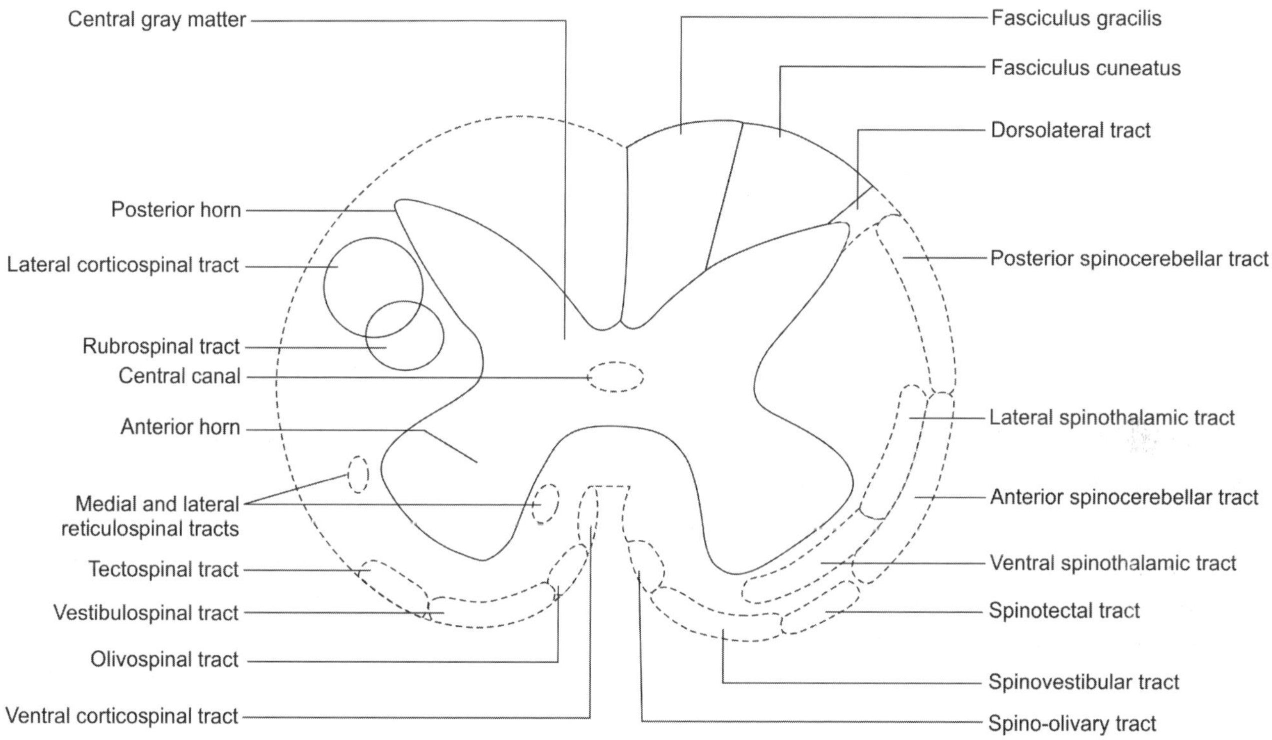

Figure 4.1: Major tracts in spinal cord—descending and ascending (*For color version, see Plate 7*)

KEY FEATURES

- Descending tracts: Can be cortical (i) or subcortical (ii–iv)
  1. Lateral and anterior corticospinal tracts—control skeletal muscles.
  2. Rubrospinal tract—part of extrapyramidal system, it facilitates flexors and inhibits extensors.
  3. Lateral reticulospinal tract—facilitates motor neurons.
  4. Medial reticulospinal tract—inhibits motor neurons.

- Ascending tracts: Carries sensation from body except head and neck.
  - Fasciculus gracilis and fasciculus cuneatus—carry conscious proprioception (sense of pressure, vibration, movement, position and fine touch).
  - Posterior spinocerebellar tract—carries unconscious proprioception from same side of the body.
  - Anterior spinocerebellar tract—carries unconscious proprioception from opposite side of the body.
  - Lateral spinothalamic tract—carries pain and temperature from opposite side of the body.
  - Anterior spinothalamic tract—carries crude touch and pressure from opposite side of the body.

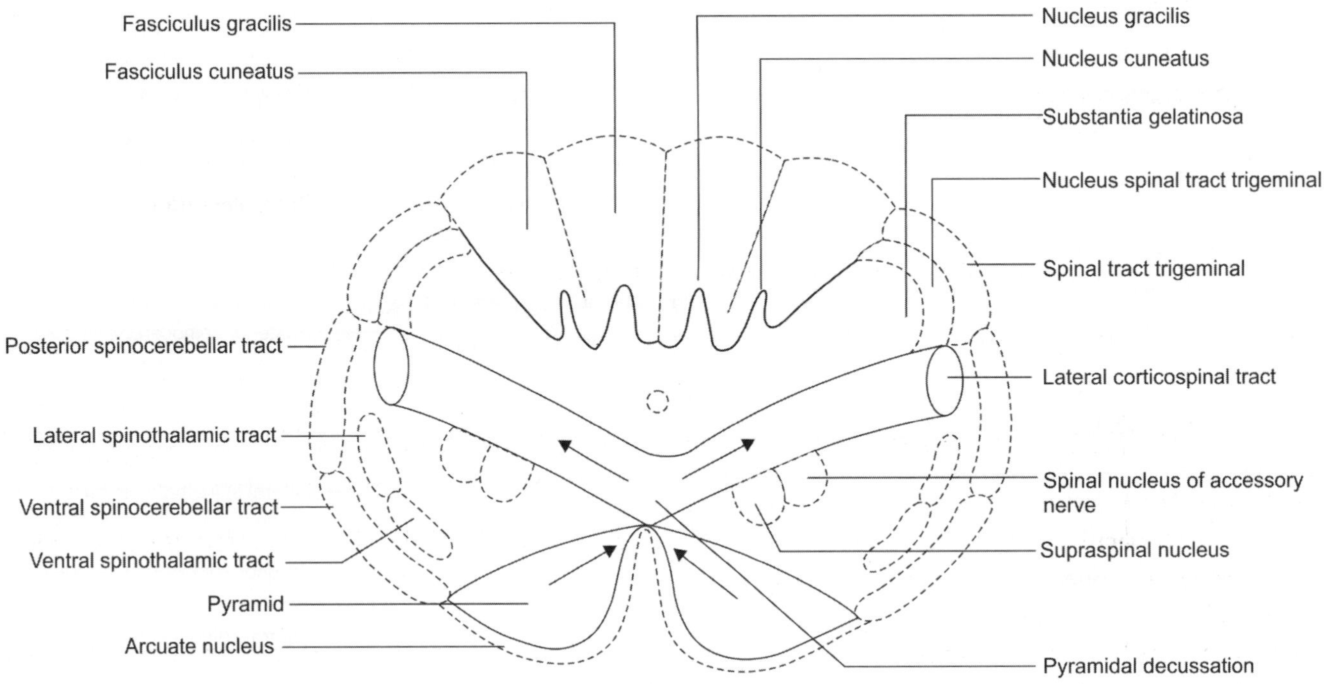

Figure 4.2: Section of medulla—pyramidal decussation (*For color version, see Plate 7*)

KEY FEATURES

- Pyramids decussate to form lateral and anterior corticospinal tracts
- Anterior horn of gray matter is replaced by supraspinal nucleus medially and spinal nucleus of accessory nerve laterally
- Tip of posterior horn along with overlying tract become spinal tract and nucleus of trigeminal nerve
- Beginning of nucleus gracilis and cuneatus.

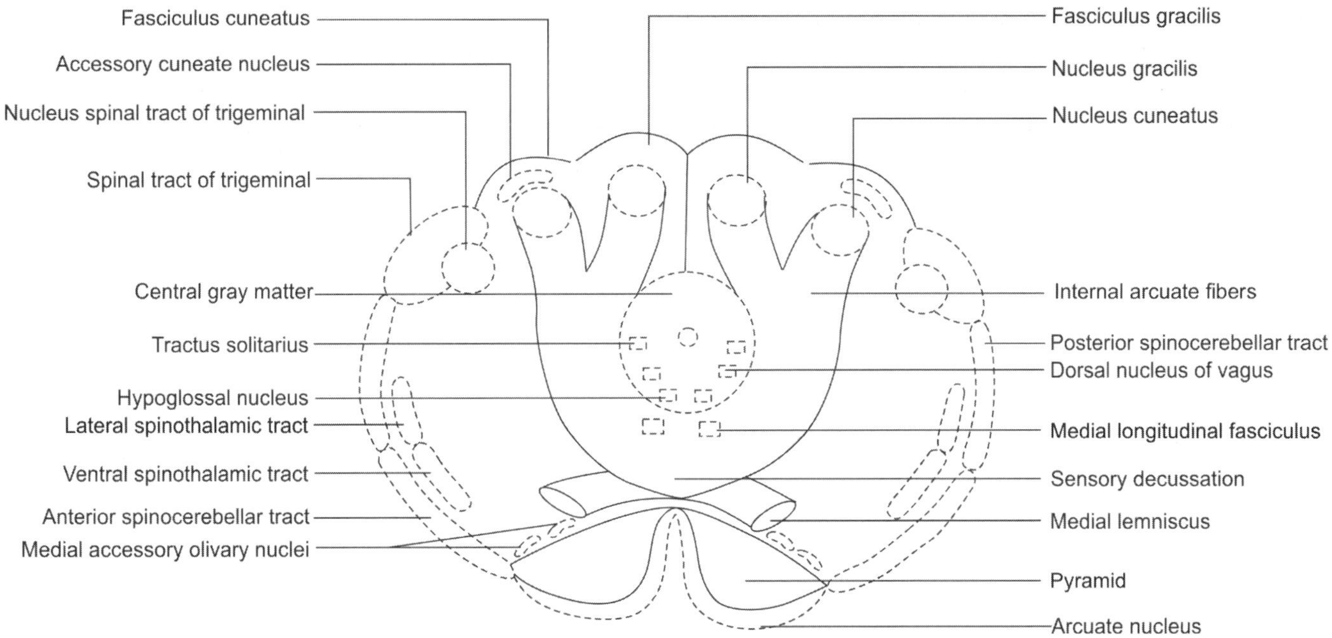

Figure 4.3: Section of medulla—sensory decussation (*For color version, see Plate 8*)

KEY FEATURES

- Accessory cuneate nucleus appears
- Fibers of fasciculus gracilis and cuneatus synapse in respective nuclei and decussate as internal arcuate fibers to form medial lemniscus
- Spinal tract and nucleus of trigeminal nerve become detached
- Gray matter becomes localized in center and following nuclei make their appearance—hypoglossal nucleus, dorsal nucleus of vagus and nucleus of tractus solitarius
- Medial longitudinal fasciculus (intersegmental tract of brainstem) appears
- Medial accessory olivary nucleus appears between decussation and pyramid.

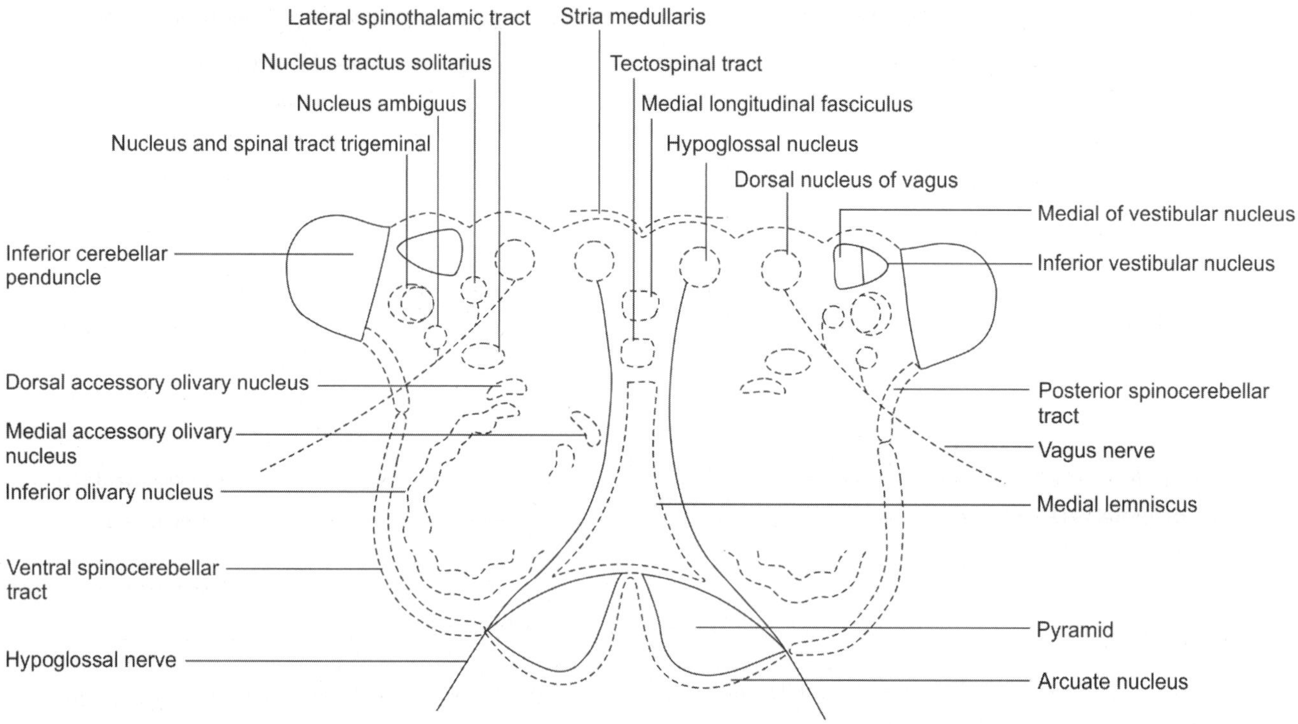

Figure 4.4: Section of medulla—inferior olivary nucleus (*For color version, see Plate 8*)

KEY FEATURES

- It lies in the floor of 4th ventricle due to the opening of central canal
- From medial to lateral side the nuclei are hypoglossal, dorsal nucleus of vagus and vestibular nuclear group
- Anterior to them are spinal tract and nucleus of 5th, nucleus ambiguus, nucleus tractus solitarius and lateral spinothalamic tract
- Laterally the posterior spinocerebellar tract enters inferior cerebellar peduncle
- Inferior cerebellar peduncle emerges from medulla to enter cerebellum
- In paramedian position are medial lemniscus, tectospinal tract and medial longitudinal fasciculus
- Just posterior to pyramid there are two inferior olivary nuclei
- Lesion of pyramid, medial lemniscus and hypoglossal nucleus causes medial medullary syndrome due to blockade of anterior spinal artery
- Lesion of dorsal nucleus of vagus, vestibular nuclei, spinal tract and nucleus of 5th, nucleus ambiguus, nucleus tractus solitarius and lateral spinothalamic tract causes lateral medullary syndrome due to blockade of posterior inferior cerebellar artery.

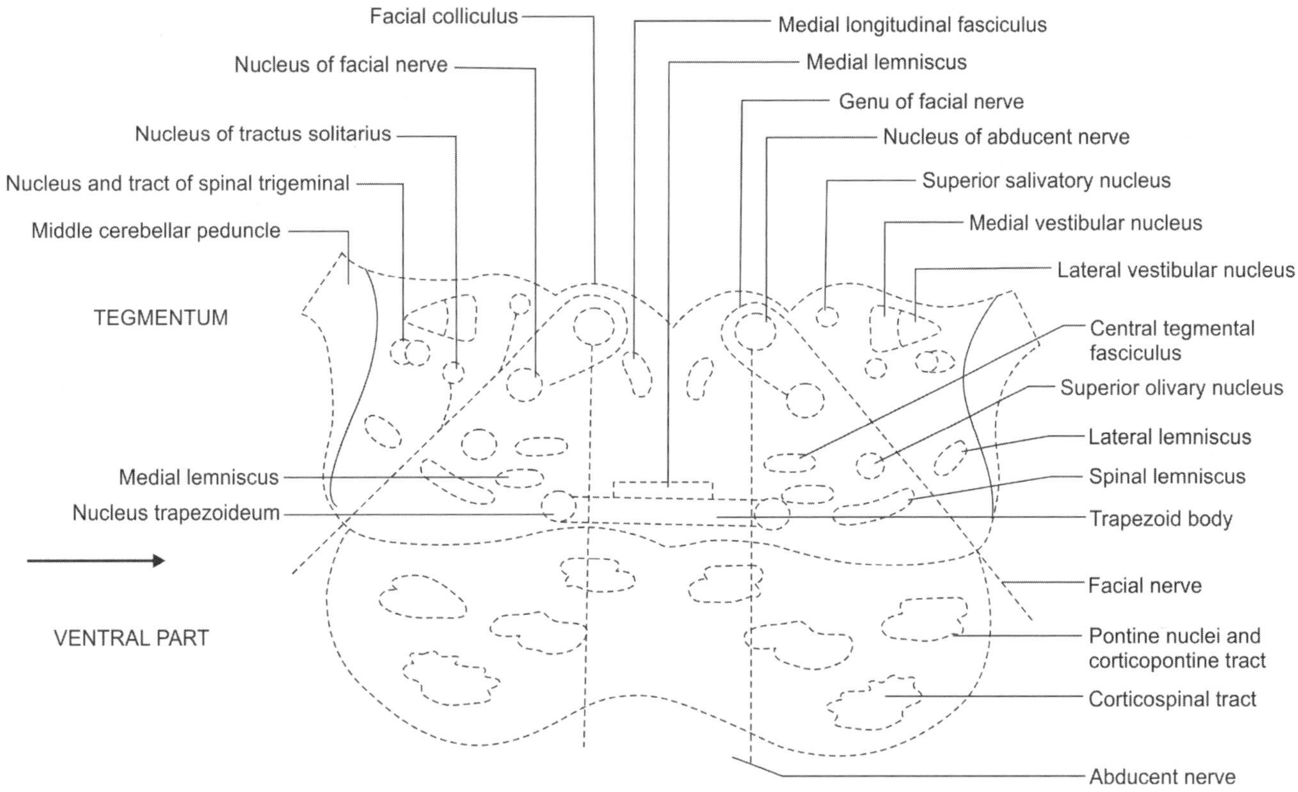

Figure 4.5: Section pons—facial colliculus

KEY FEATURES

- Ventral part is related to basilar artery and contains scattered nuclei pontis, corticopontine, corticonuclear and corticospinal tracts
- Close to the ventral part following structures are arranged from median to lateral side—medial, trigeminal, spinal and lateral lemnisci
- Medial lemniscus carries conscious proprioception, trigeminal lemniscus carries pain and temperature from head and neck, spinal lemniscus carries pain and temperature from rest of the body and lateral lemniscus formed at this level carries auditory information
- Fibers from facial nucleus wind around abducent nucleus to form an elevation in the floor of 4th ventricle called facial colliculus
- Laterally middle cerebellar peduncle arises from pons to enter cerebellum. It contains crossed pontocerebellar fibers.

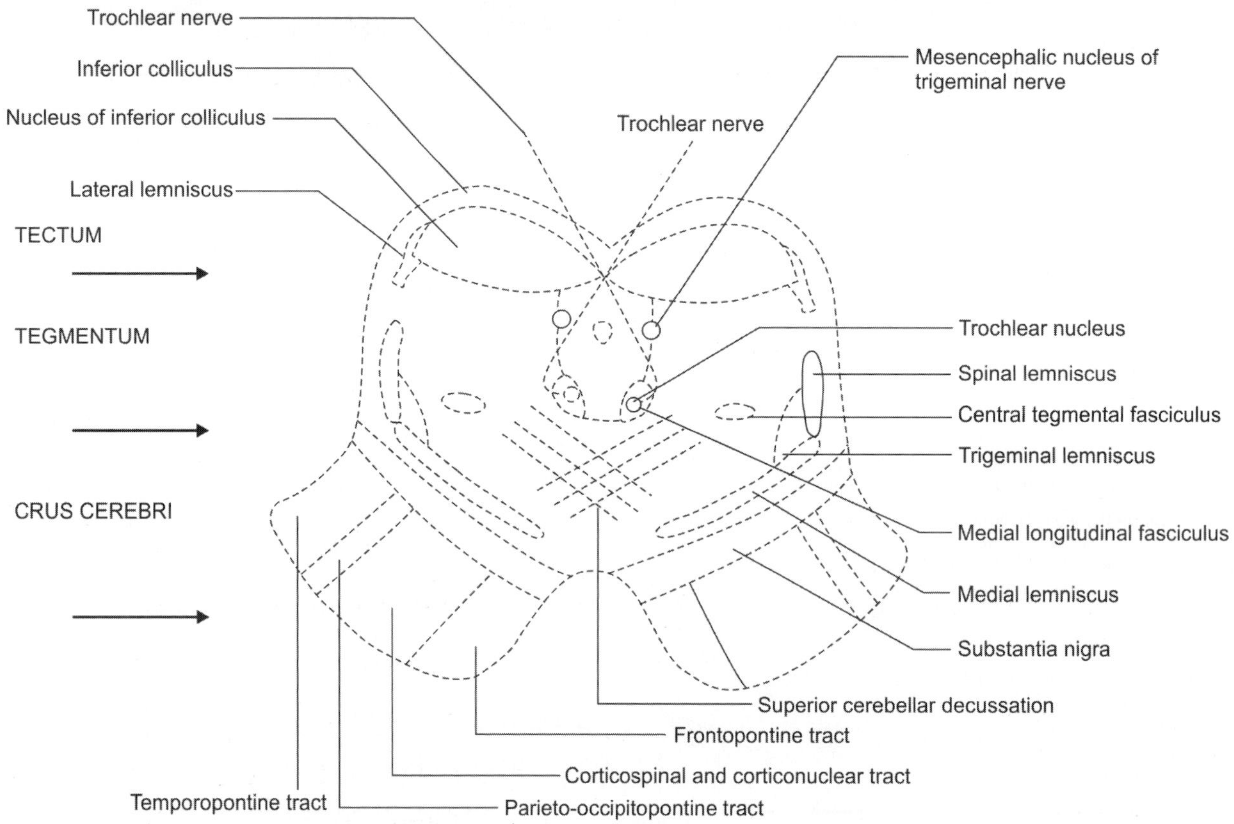

Figure 4.6: Section midbrain—inferior colliculus

KEY FEATURES

- Internally it is divided into three parts—crus cerebri, tegmentum and tectum:
  i. Crus cerebri is essentially made up of projection fibers which emerge from cerebrum. It is made up of corticospinal, corticonuclear and corticopontine fibers. It is separated from tegmentum by substantia nigra.
  ii. Tegmentum contains medial, trigeminal and spinal lemnisci. The lateral lemniscus enters inferior colliculus. Central gray contains trochlear and mesencephalic nuclei. Ventral to the gray matter there is decussation of superior cerebellar peduncle.
  iii. Tectum is entirely made up of inferior colliculus which is the auditory relay center.

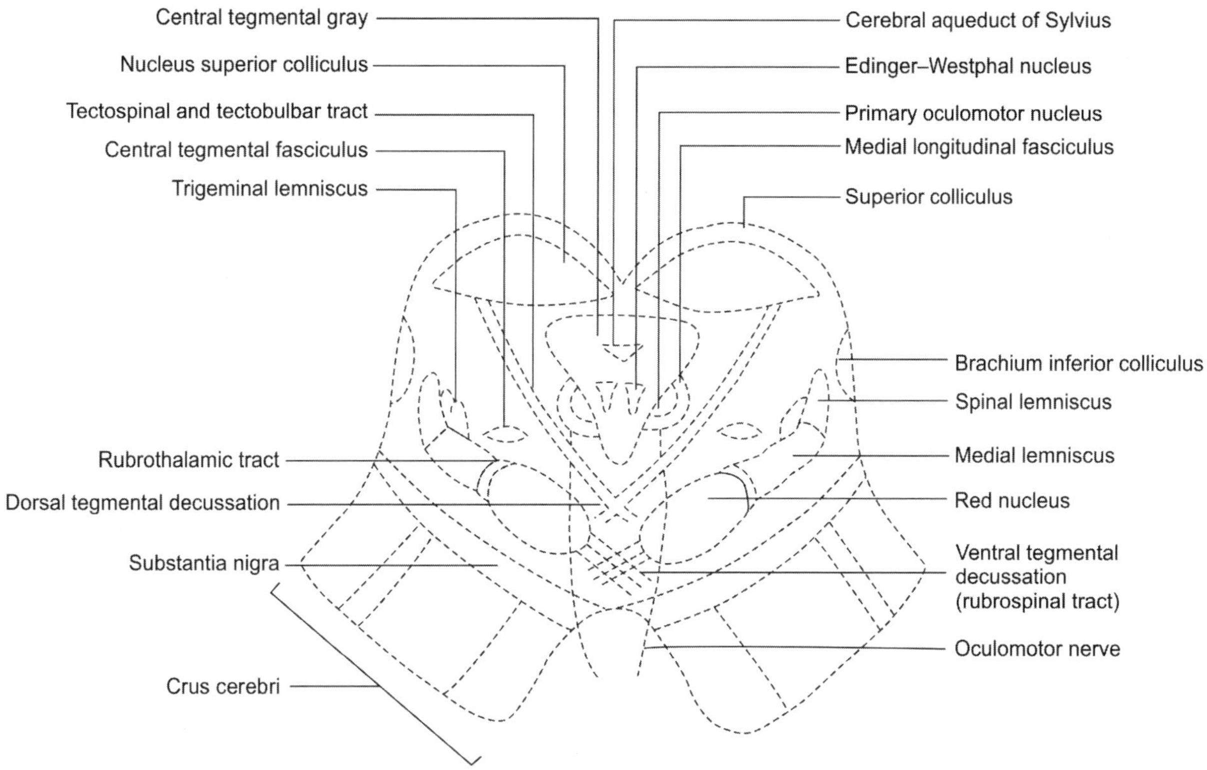

Figure 4.7: Section midbrain—superior colliculus

KEY FEATURES

- Crus cerebri has same composition as at inferior collicular level
- Tegmentum—red nucleus appears in which the fibers of superior cerebellar peduncle synapse and ascend as rubrothalamic tract. Ventral tegmental decussation is formed by rubrospinal tract and dorsal tegmental decussation is formed by tectospinal tract. Gray matter shows occulomotor and Edinger-Westphal nucleus
- Tectum is entirely made up of superior colliculus which is the visual relay center.

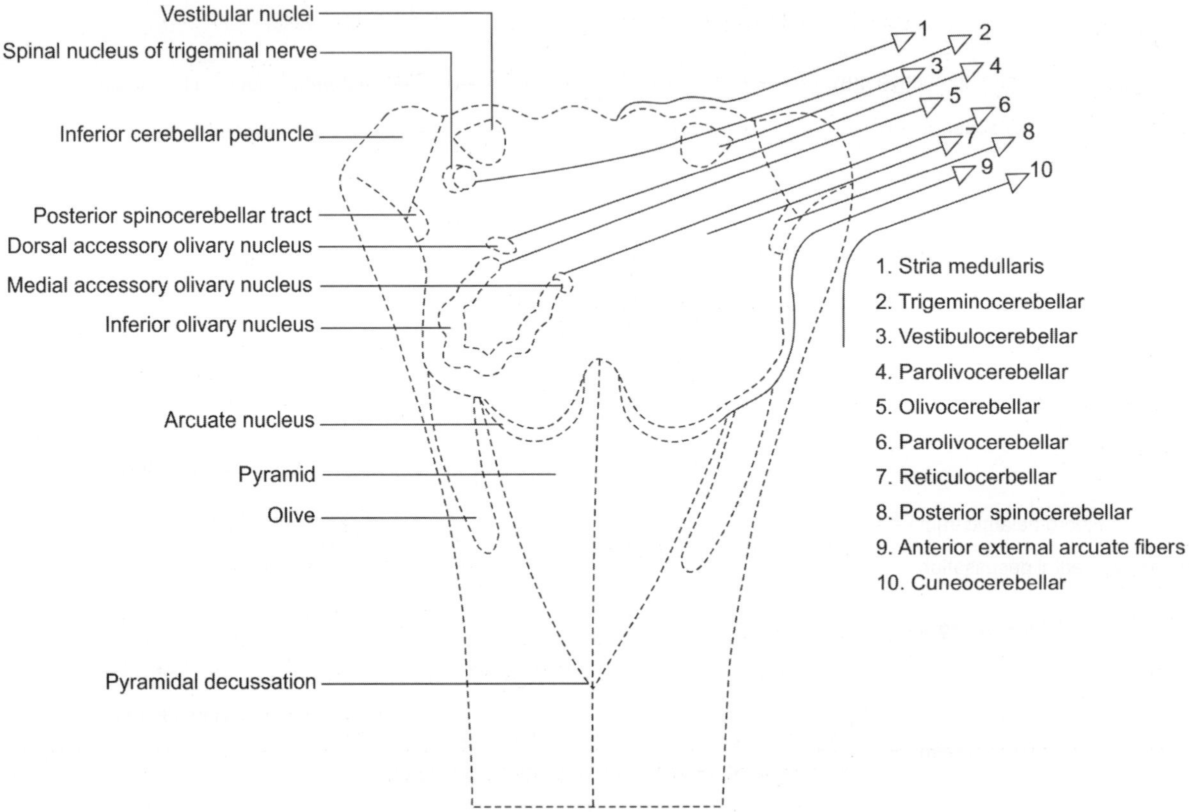

Figure 4.8: Inferior cerebellar peduncle—afferent fibers

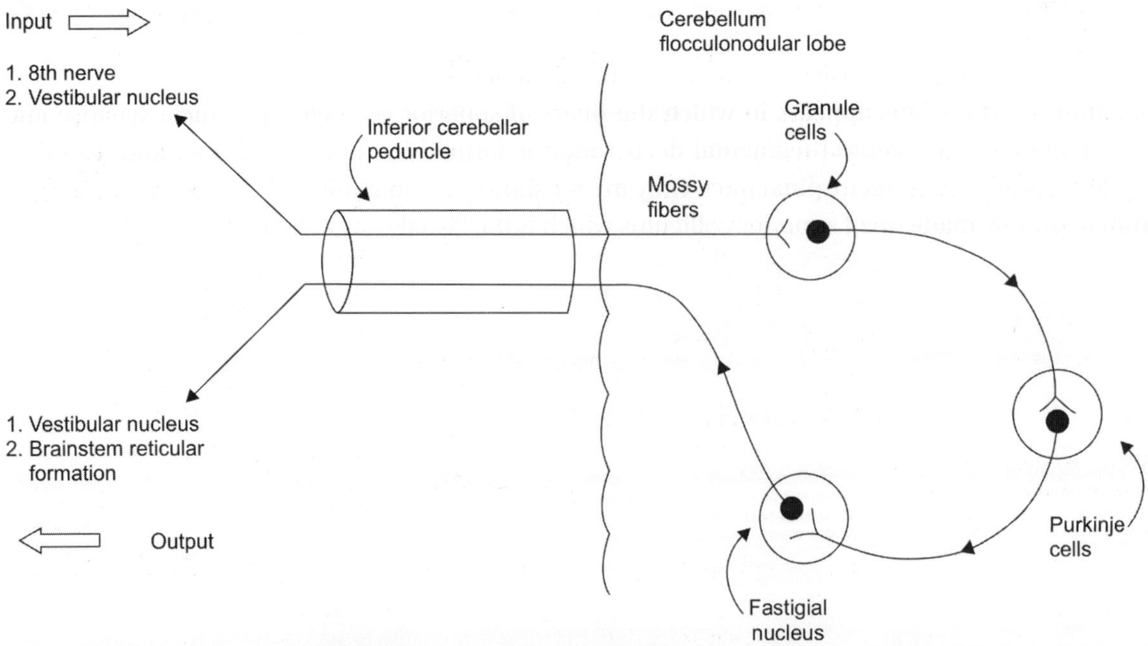

Figure 4.9: Vestibular-archicerebellar connections

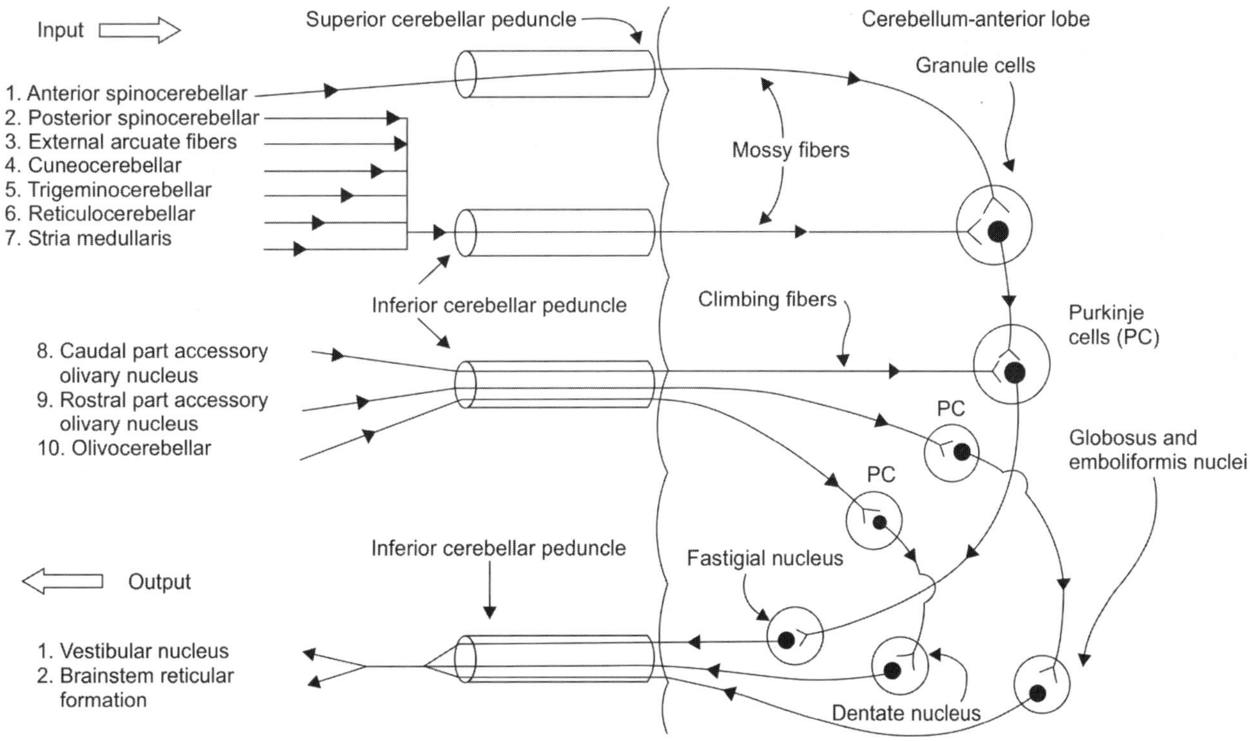

Figure 4.10: Spinal-paleocerebellar connections

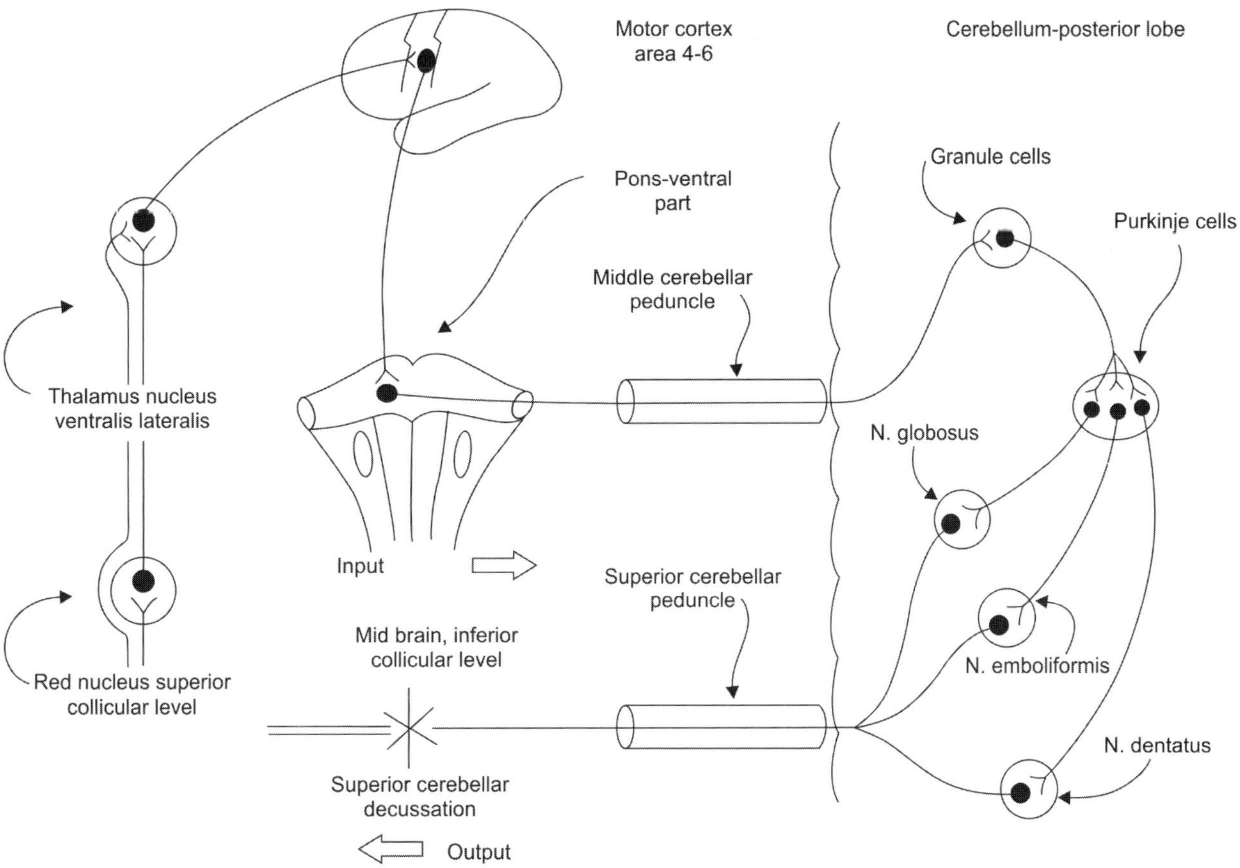

Figure 4.11: Cortical-neocerebellar connections

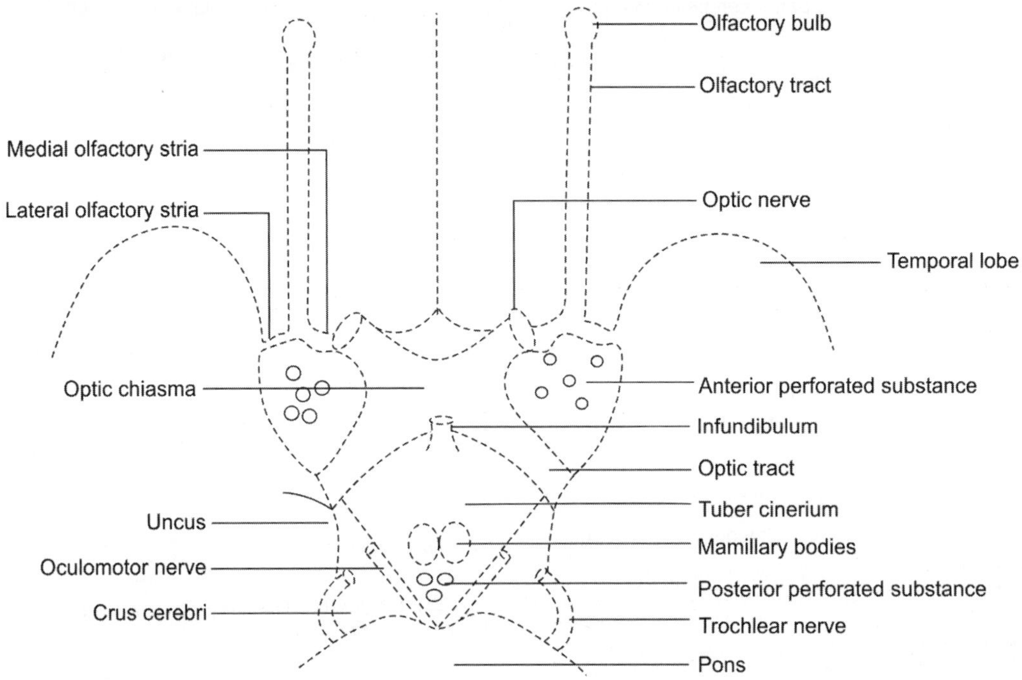

Figure 4.12: Interpeduncular fossa

KEY FEATURES

- It is an area on the ventral aspect of brain between two temporal lobes
- Anteriorly—optic chiasma. Posteriorly—Pons
- Anterolaterally—optic tract. Posterolaterally—crus cerebri
- It has following structures arranged anteroposteriorly—infundibulum, tuber cinerium, mamillary bodies and posterior perforated substance. These structures separate cavity of 3rd ventricle from Interpeduncular cistern. Occulomotor nerve emerges from the medial aspect of crus cerebri.

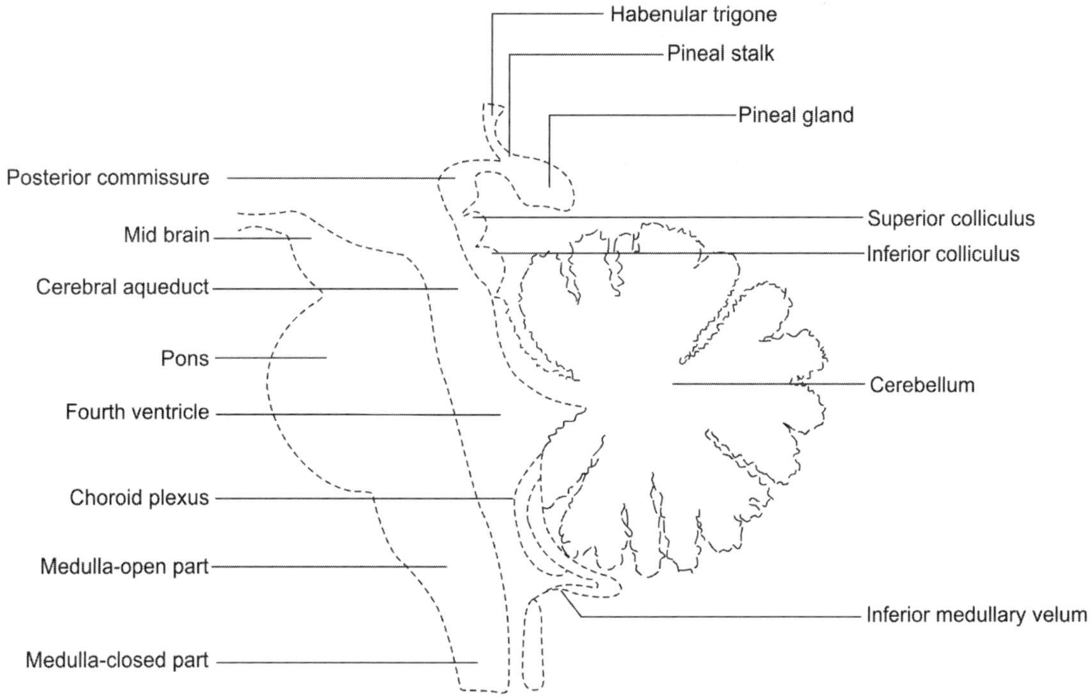

Figure 4.13: Fourth ventricle—sagittal section

KEY FEATURES

- Triangular in shape in sagittal section. Above it continues as cerebral aqueduct.
- Below continues as central canal. Its apex extends into cerebellum as median dorsal recess.
- The roof is separated from cerebellum by superior and inferior medullary velum.
- It communicates with subarachnoid space through two lateral recesses and one median dorsal recess
- The choroid plexus invaginates in 4th ventricle.

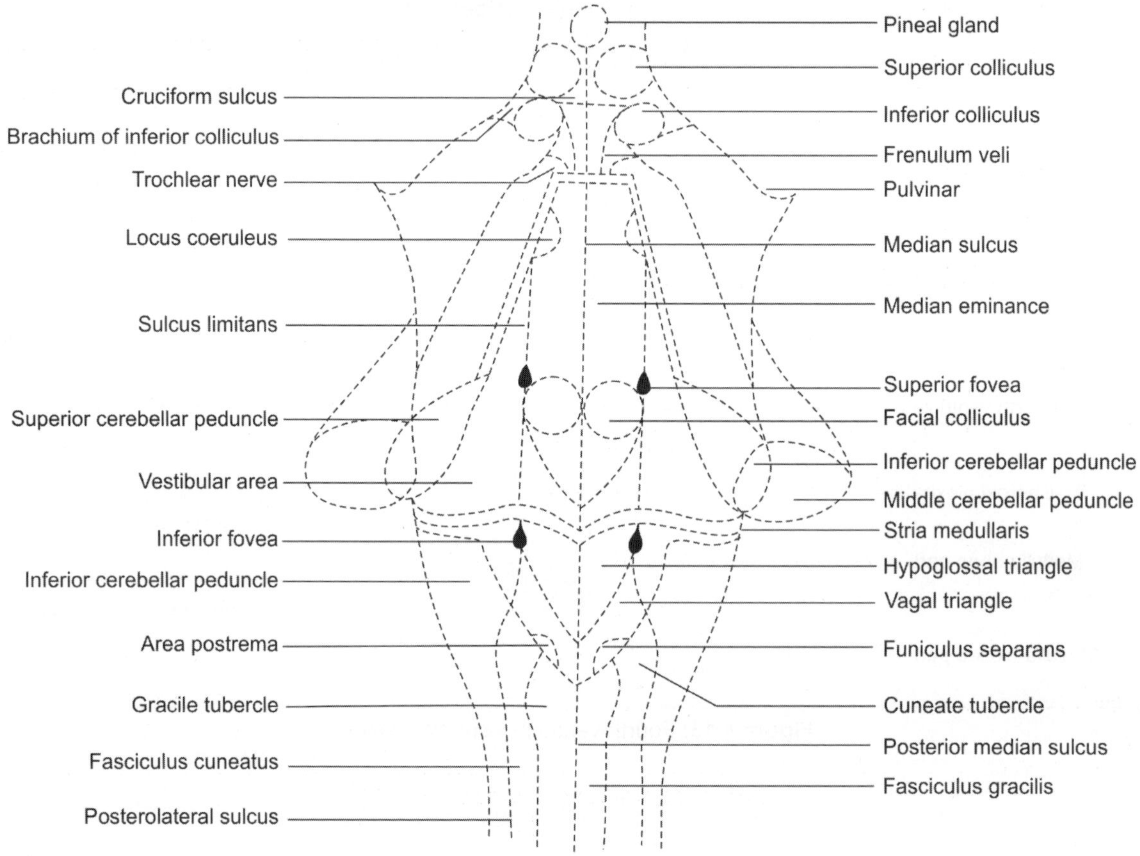

Figure 4.14: Floor of 4th ventricle

KEY FEATURES

- Formed by dorsal aspect pons and open part medulla
- It is rhomboid in shape
- It has a median sulcus and two paramedian sulci called sulcus limitans having superior and inferior fovea
- Paramedian area above downwards has—locus coeruleus, facial colliculus, stria medullaris, hypoglossal triangle, vagal triangle and area postrema
- Lateral to sulcus limitans there is triangular vestibular area.

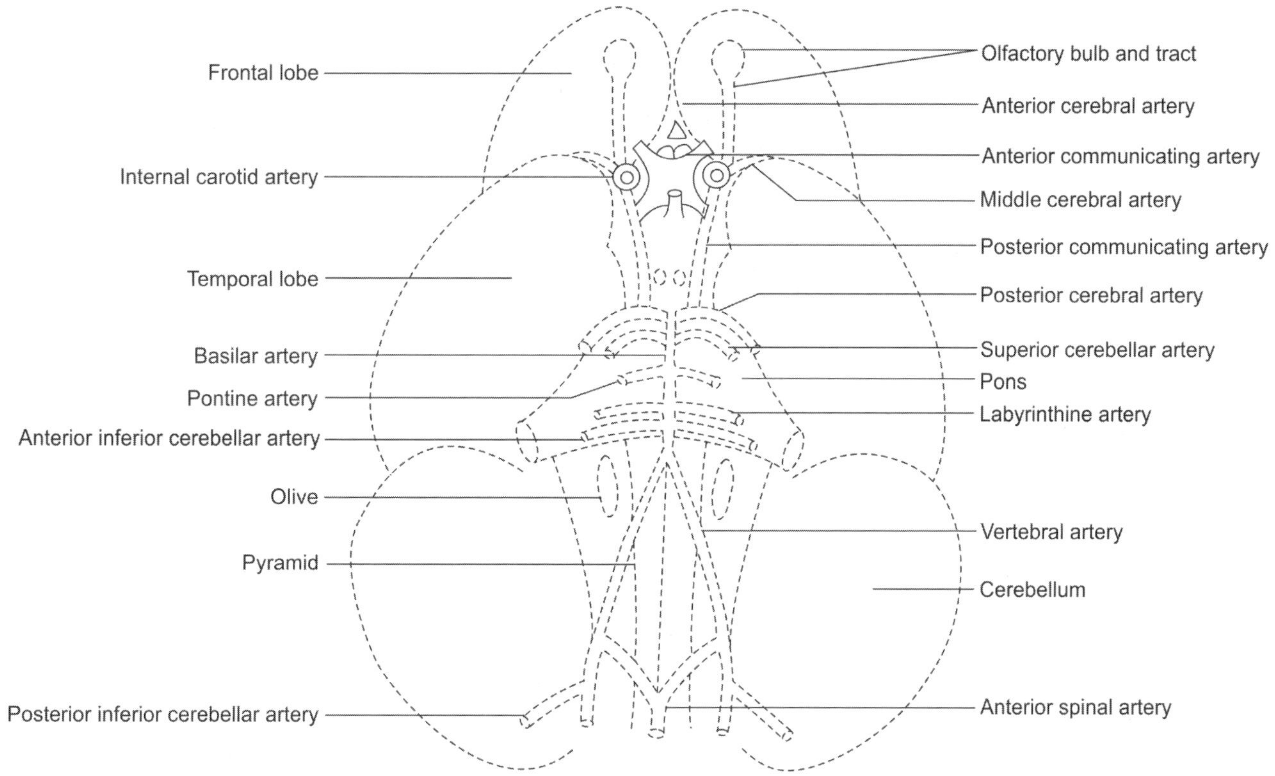

Figure 4.15: Arteries on the base of brain

KEY FEATURES

- Brain is supplied by internal carotid and vertebrobasilar system of arteries
- Internal carotid artery enters skull through foramen lacerum, traverses cavernous sinus and reaches base of brain lateral to optic chiasma
- Internal carotid artery divides into:
  - Anterior cerebral artery enters longitudinal fissure and communicates with opposite artery.
  - Middle cerebral artery enters lateral sulcus of brain.
  - Posterior communicating artery communicates with posterior cerebral artery.
- Vertebrobasilar system—two vertebral arteries enter skull through foramen magnum, unite to form basilar artery at pontomedullary junction. Then runs ventral to pons and divides in two terminal branches—posterior cerebral arteries.
- Other branches given off are:
  - Anterior spinal.
  - Posterior inferior cerebellar.
  - Anterior inferior cerebellar.
  - Labyrinthine.
  - Pontine.
  - Superior cerebellar.

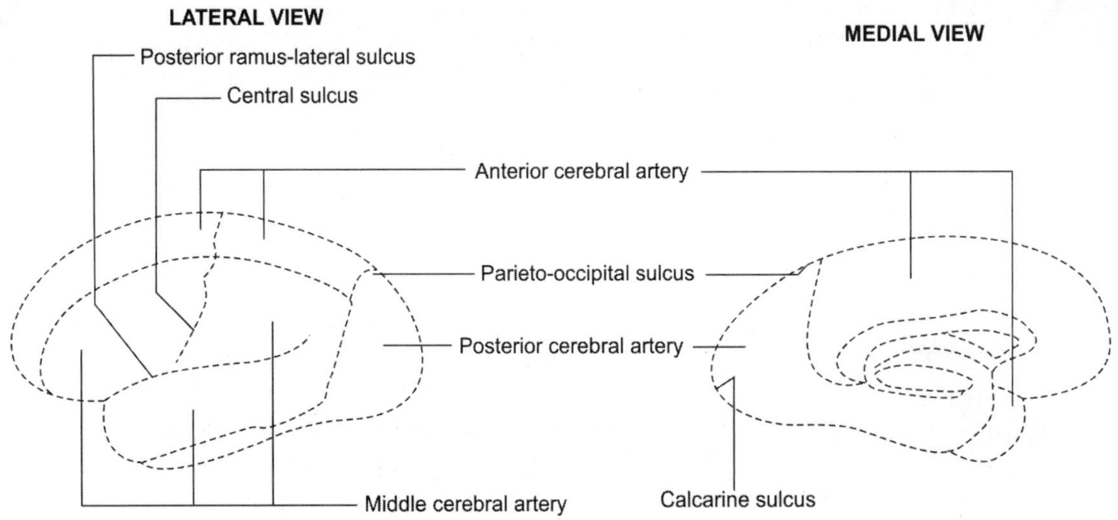

Figure 4.16: Areas of blood supply—brain

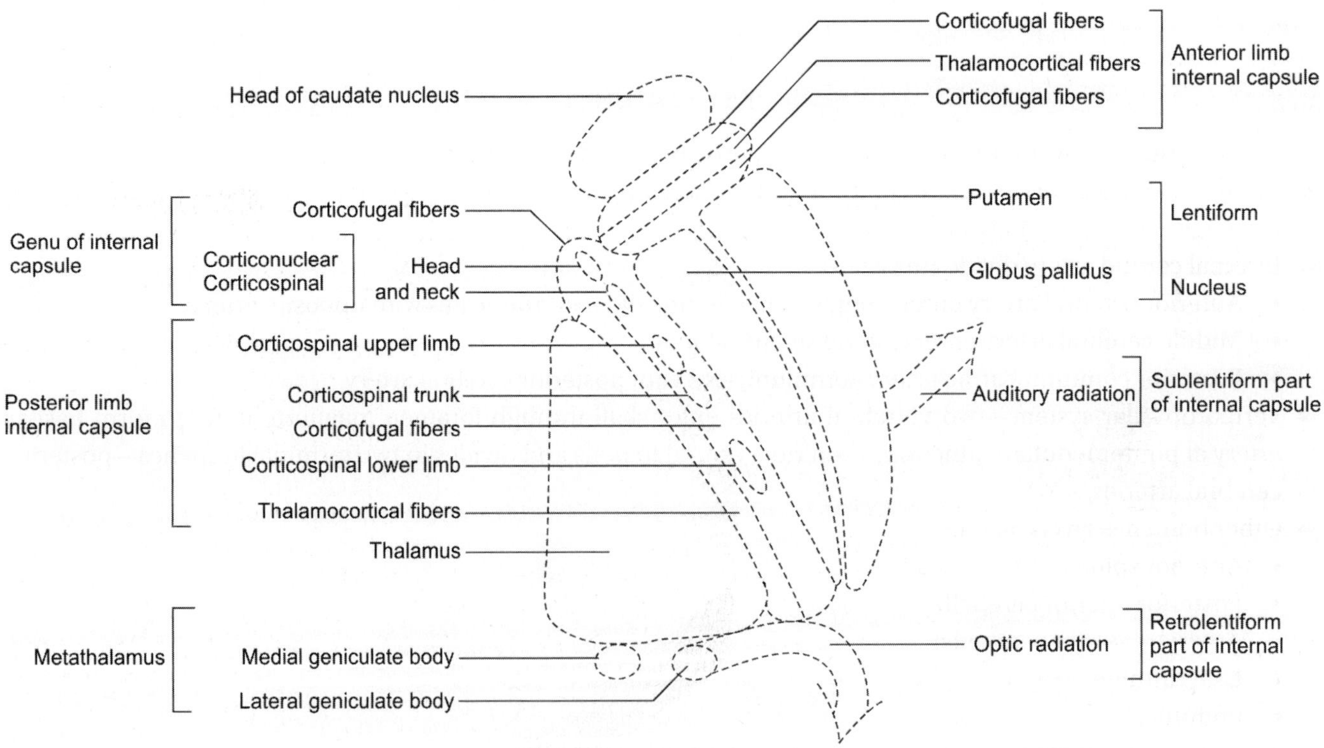

Figure 4.17: Internal capsule

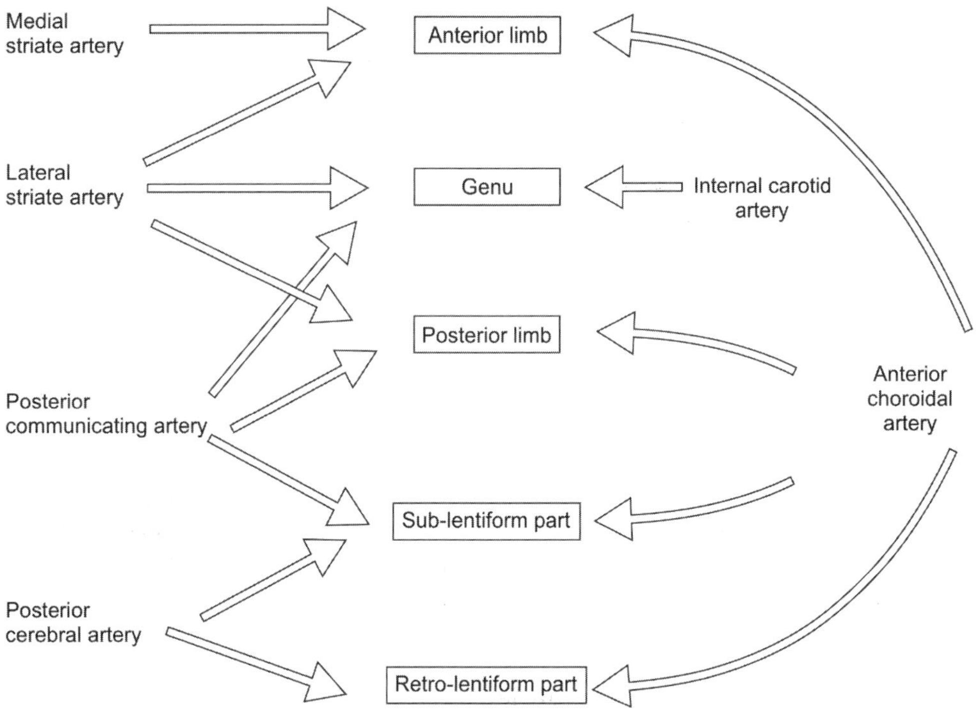

Figure 4.18: Blood supply—internal capsule

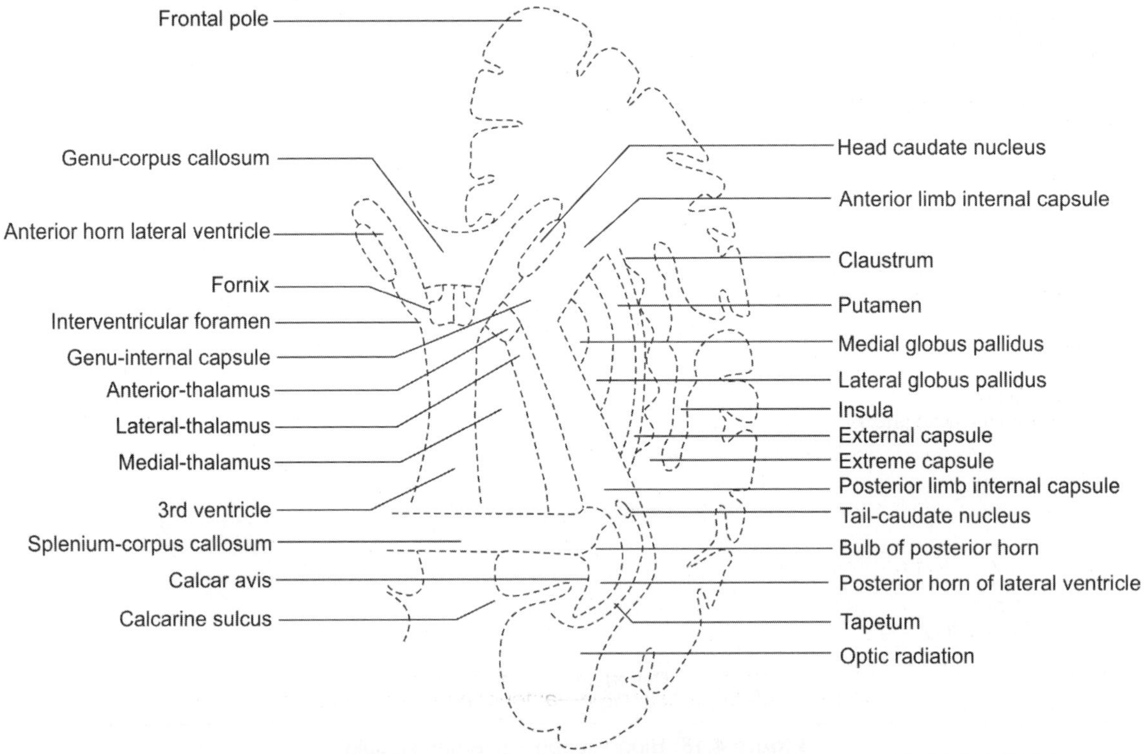

Figure 4.19: Horizontal section cerebrum—interventricular foramen

KEY FEATURES

- From lateral to medial side following structures are seen:
  - Lateral sulcus
  - Insula
  - Insular cortex
  - Extreme capsule
  - Claustrum
  - External capsule
  - Putamen
  - Globus pallidus lateral
  - Globus pallidus medial
  - Internal capsule
  - Head of caudate nucleus (anteriorly) and hypothalamus (posteriorly)
  - 3rd ventricle.
- Two cerebral hemispheres are connected by commissural fibers
- Biggest bundle of commissural fibers is corpus callosum
- It has following parts—rostrum, genu, body and splenium
- Posterior part of body and anterior part of splenium form tapetum.

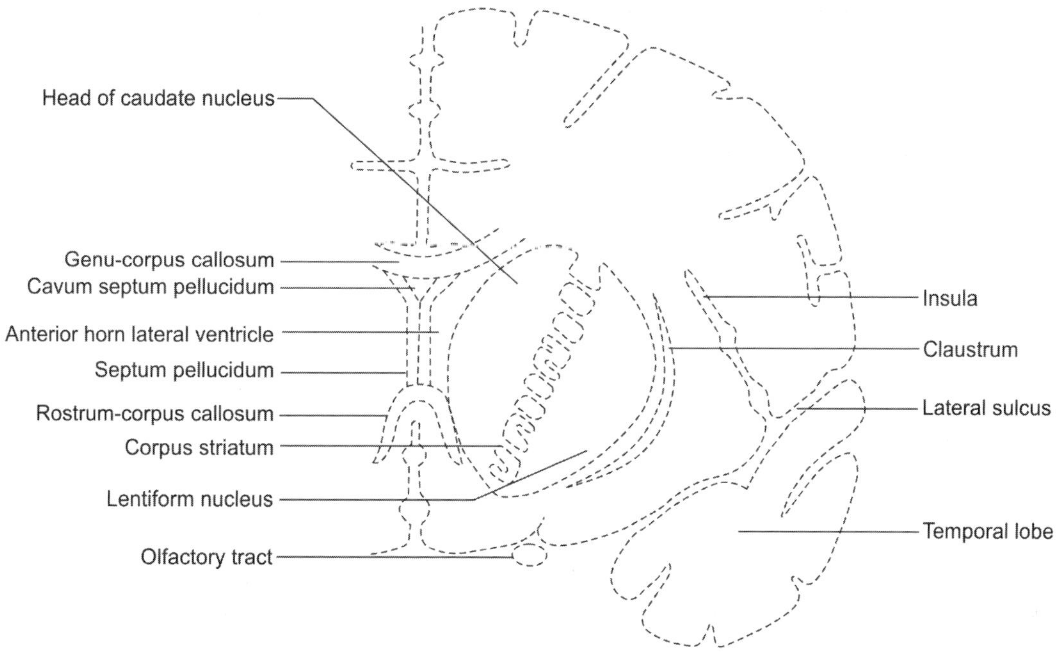

Figure 4.20: Coronal section—anterior horn lateral ventricle

KEY FEATURES

- Medial wall—septum pellucidum and rostrum of corpus callosum
- Floor—head of the caudate nucleus
- Roof—corpus callosum
- Anterior end—genu of corpus callosum.

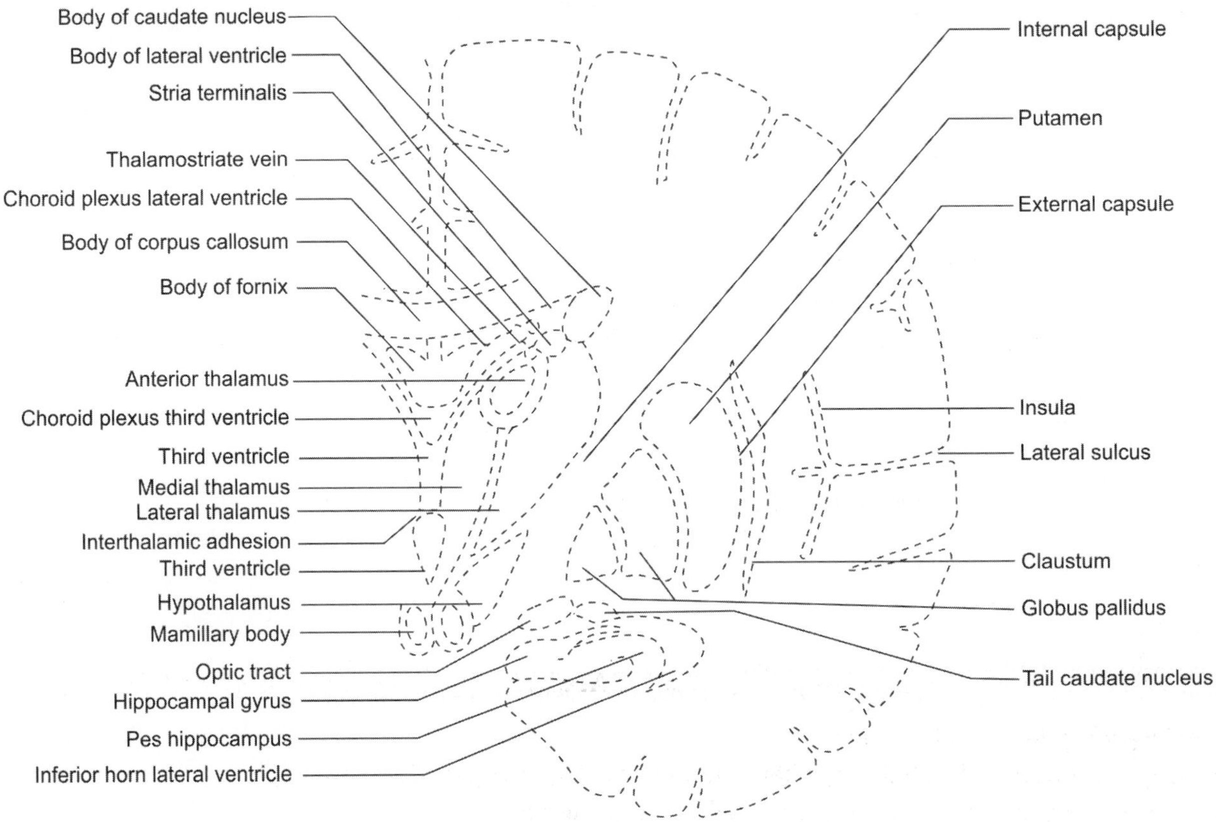

Figure 4.21: Coronal section—body of lateral ventricle

KEY FEATURES

This section depicts body and inferior horn of lateral ventricle.

- Body:
  - Medial wall—body of fornix.
  - Floor—from medial to lateral side:
    - Superior surface thalamus, lateral part
    - Thalamostriate vein
    - Stria terminalis
    - Body of the caudate nucleus.
  - Roof—corpus callosum.
- Inferior horn:
  - Floor—pes hippocampus medially and collateral eminence laterally.
  - Roof and lateral wall—tapetum.

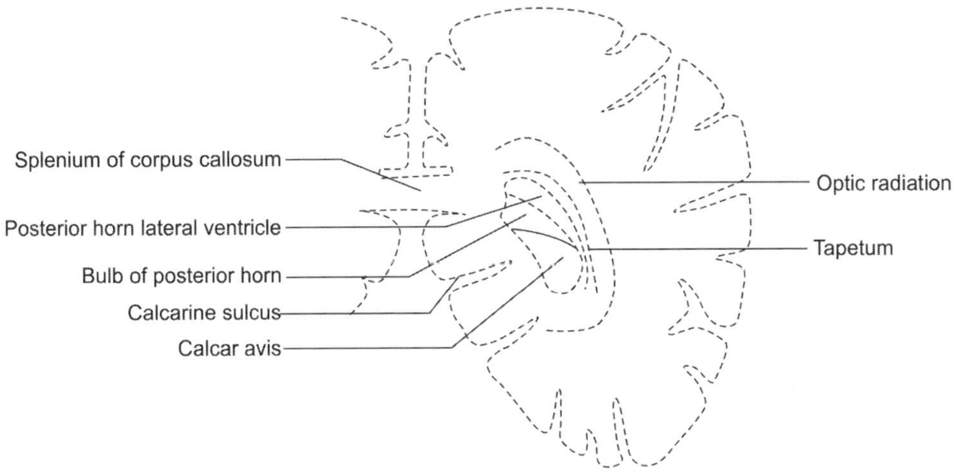

Figure 4.22: Coronal section—posterior horn lateral ventricle

KEY FEATURES

- Medial wall shows two elevations:
  - Upper elevation called bulb of posterior horn caused by forceps major (part of splenium of corpus callosum)
  - Lower elevation called calcar avis caused by calcarine sulcus.
- Roof and lateral wall—tapetum which separates the posterior horn from optic radiation.

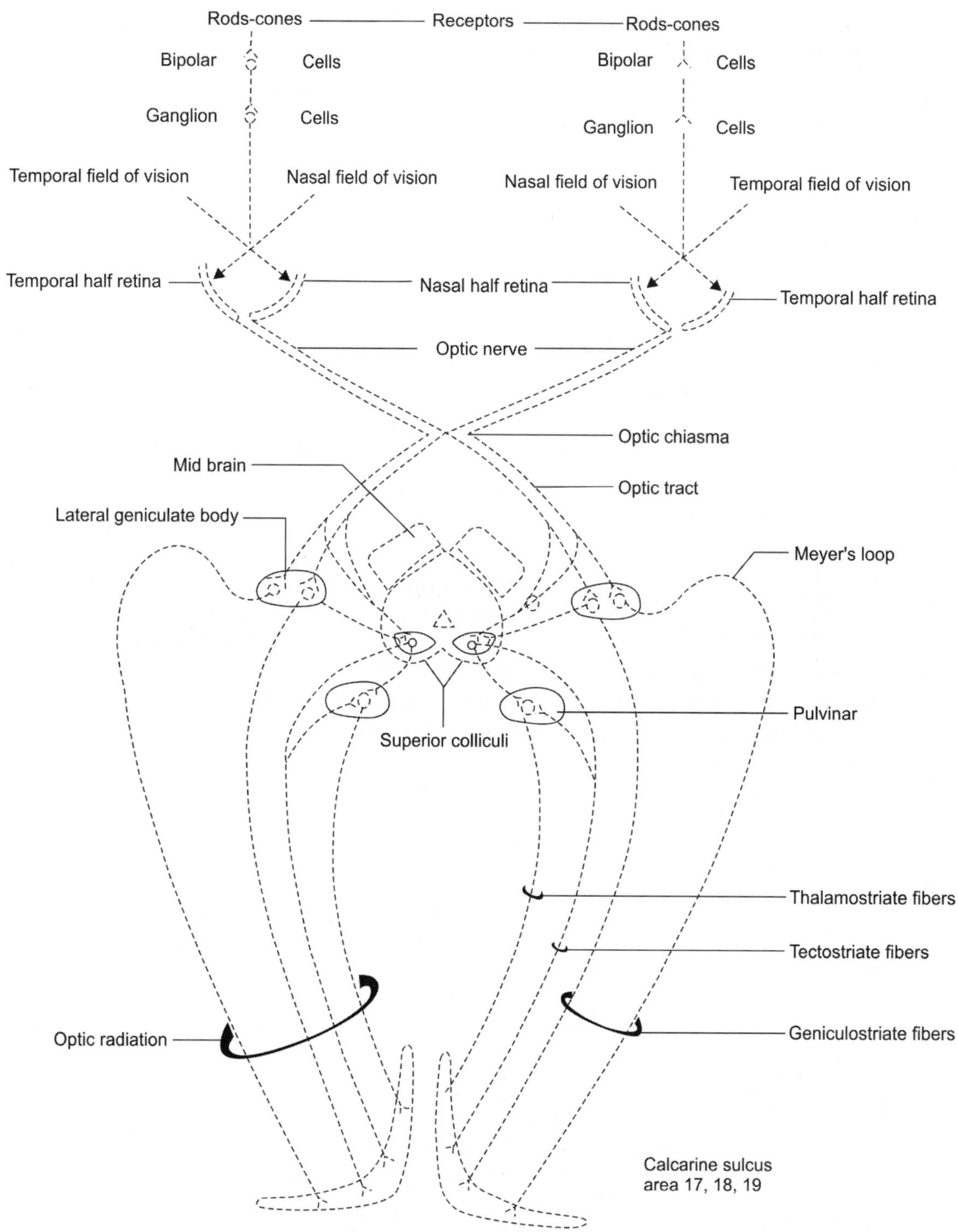

Figure 4.23: Visual pathway

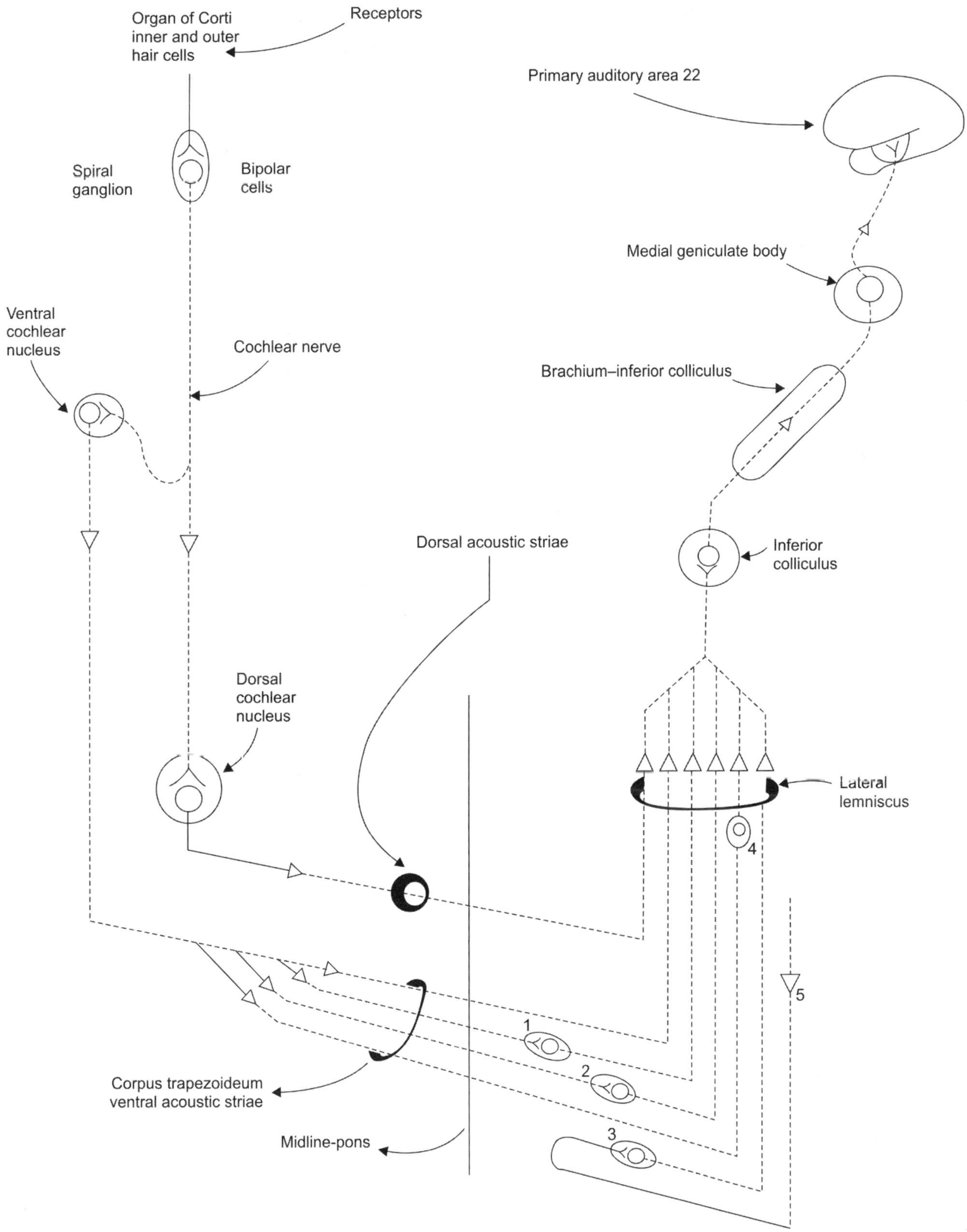

Figure 4.24: Auditory pathway: 1—NUC of corpus trapezoideum; 2,3—superior olivary complex; 4—NUC of lateral lemniscus; 5—ipsilateral fibers ventral cochlear nucleus

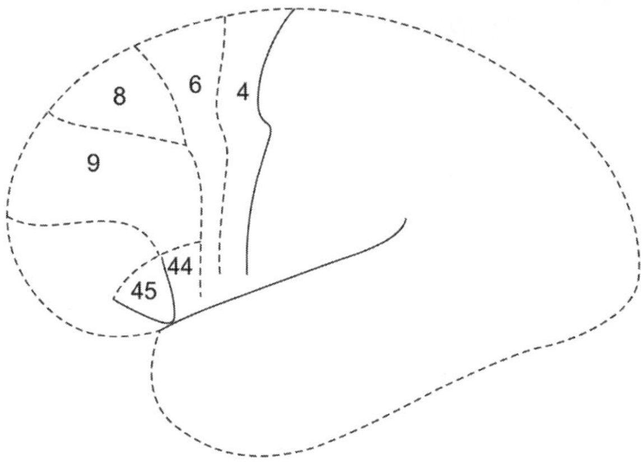

Area 4= Precentral gyrus—general movement control; Areas 6-8-9 = Premotor—some general movement control-connections to basal ganglia-controls eye movements; Areas 44-45 = Brocas area—speech movements

Figure 4.25: Brain-lateral view—motor functions

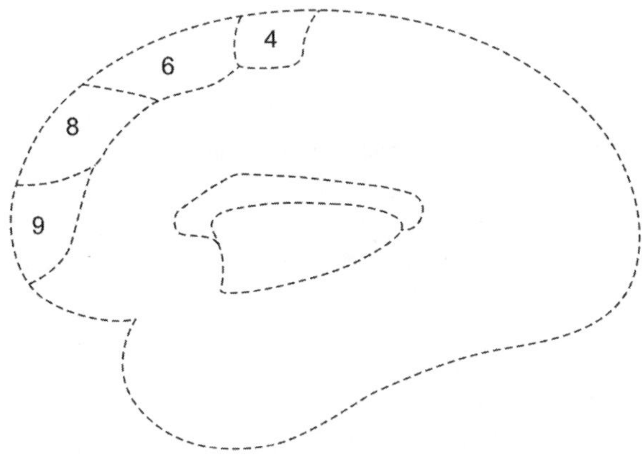

Area 4 = Precentral gyrus—leg and foot movements
Areas 6,8,9 = Premotor - some general movements, connections to basal ganglia

Figure 4.26: Brain-medial view—motor functions

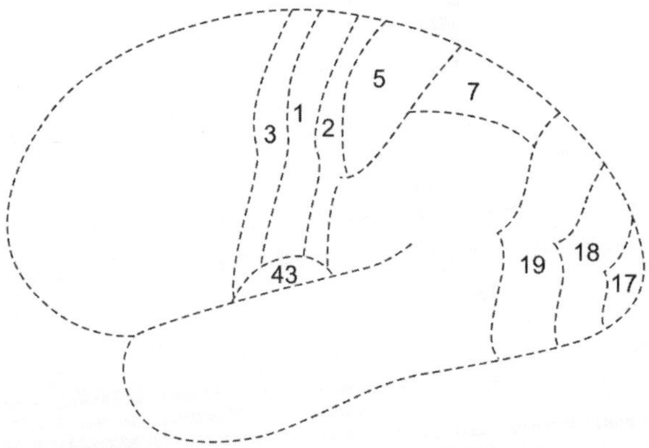

Areas 3,1,2=Postcentral gyrus—touch, pain, temperature. Conscious proprioception; Areas 5,7 = Parietal lobe—interpretation of senses perceived by 3,1,2; Area 43 = Most inferior part of postcentral gyrus—taste; Area 17 = Lips of calcarine sulcus—vision; Areas 18,19 = Rest of occipital lobe—visual interpretation area

Figure 4.27: Brain-lateral view—sensory functions

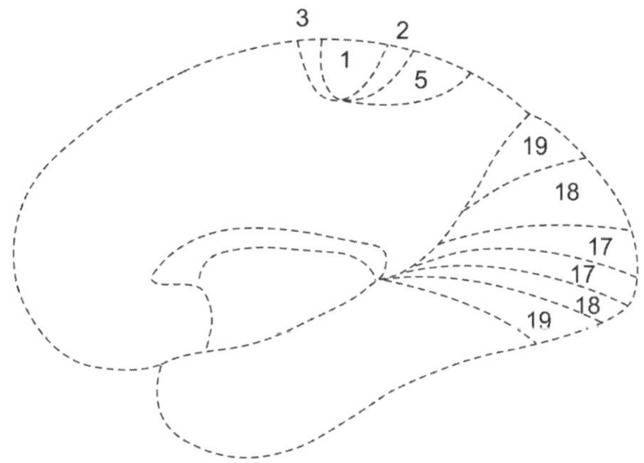

Area 3,1,2 = Postcentral gyrus—touch pain-temperature-conscious proprioception
Area 5 = Parietal lobe-interpretation of senses perceived in areas 3,1,2
Area 17 = Lips of calcarine sulcus—vision
Areas 18,19 = Rest of occipital lobe—visual interpretation area
Figure 4.28: Brain-medial view—sensory functions

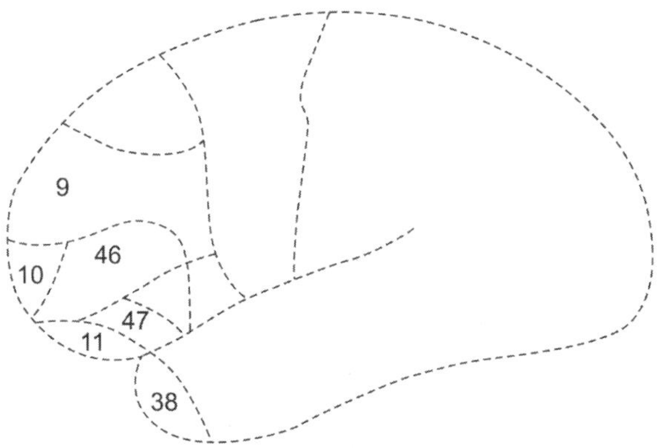

Areas 9-10-11-46-47 = Upper and anterior part—superior, middle and Inferior frontal gyri—higher intellectual functions
Area 38 = Anterior pole of temporal lobe—complex memory and imaging processes
Figure 4.29: Brain-lateral view—limbic functions

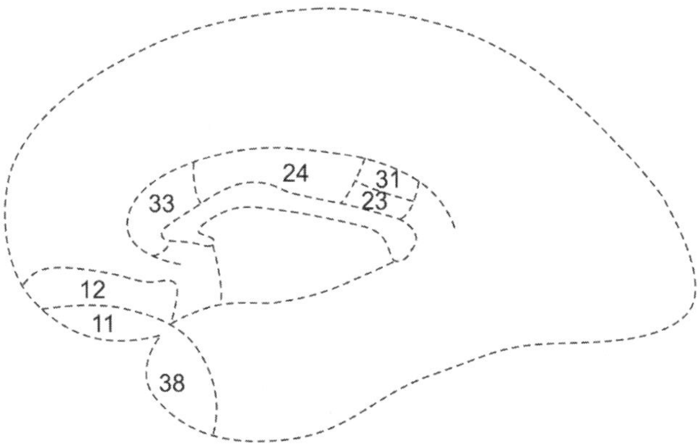

Areas 23, 24, 31, 33 = Cingulate gyrus—adds emotional tone to sensory experience including pain
Areas 11-12 = Orbital region frontal lobe—inhibitory effect on expression of emotions
Area 38 = Anterior pole temporal lobe—complex memory and imaging processes
Figure 4.30: Brain-medial view—limbic functions

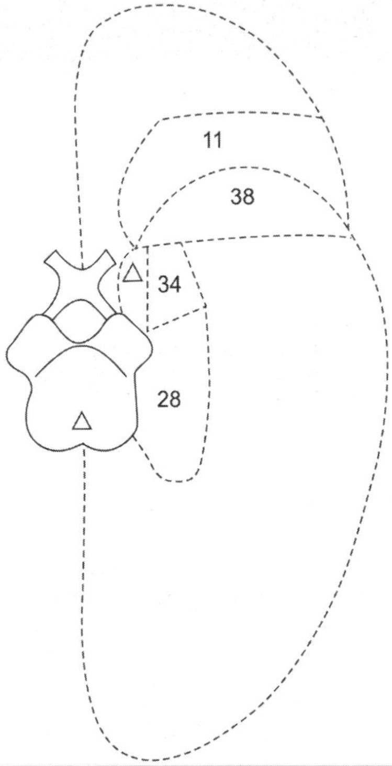

Δ - Uncus - olfactory
Area 28 = anterior part-para hippocampal
Gyrus - olfactory - memory
Area 34 - lateral to uncus - olfactory
Area 38 - arterior pole - temporal lobe-complex memory and imaging processes
Figure 4.31: Brain-basal view—olfactory and limbic functions

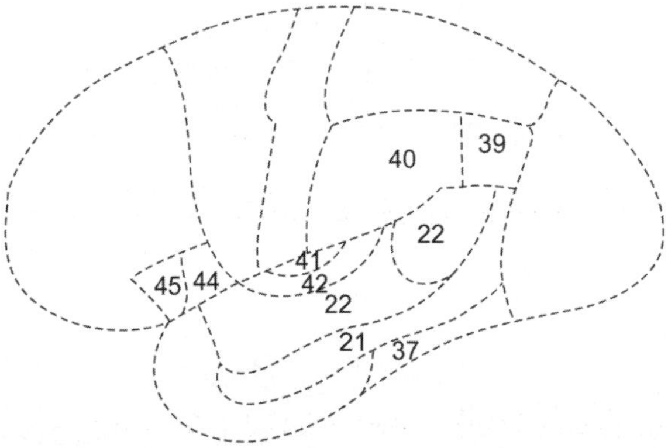

Area 41-42 = Middle of superior temporal gyrus - primary auditory, perception of sound
Area 22 = Superior temporal gyrus - Part of middle temporal gyrus - interpretation of sound including speech
Area 44-45 = Pars triangularis and opercularis - Brocas area for speech - motor
Area 22 - Posterior end superior temporal gyrus - Wernicke's area for speech - sensory
Area 39 - Angular gyrus - reading
Area 40 - Supramarginal gyrus - Understand and ability to repeat speech
Area 21 - Middle temporal gyrus - auditory memory
Area 37 - Between temporal and occipital lobes - visual memory
Figure 4.32: Brain-lateral view—hearing and language

CHAPTER 5

Thorax

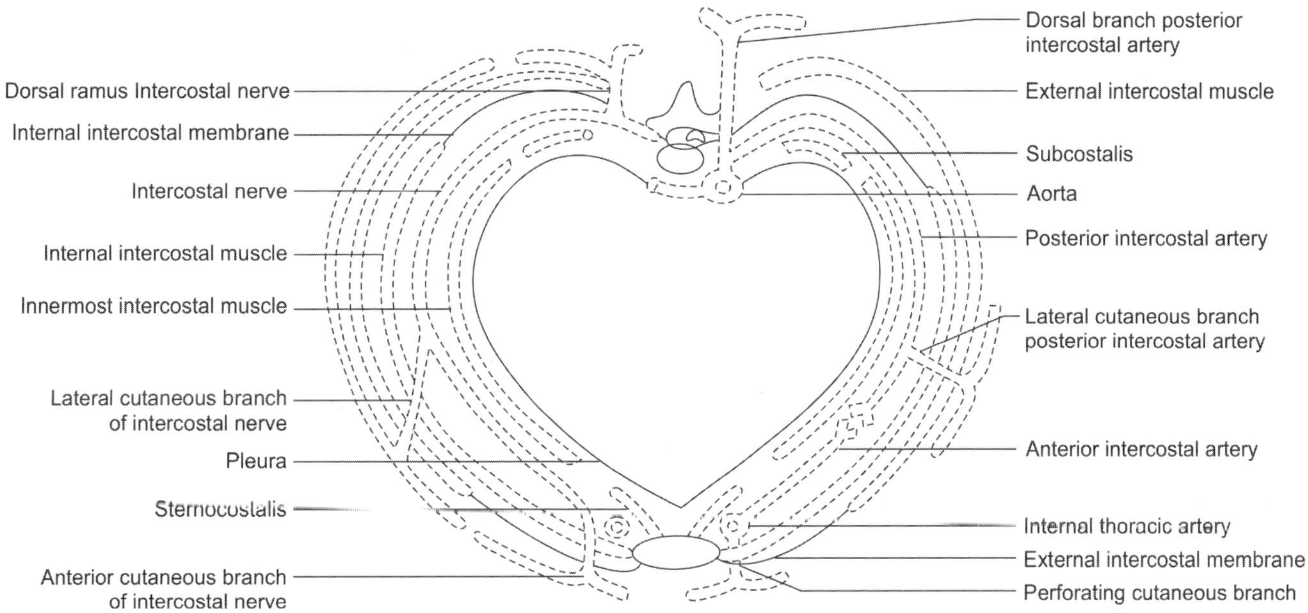

Figure 5.1: Intercostal vessels and nerves (*For color version, see Plate 9*)

KEY FEATURES

Intercostal spaces contain intercostal nerve, vein and arteries.

- Intercostal nerves: 11 in number, ventral rami of spinal nerves, do not form plexuses and are segmental in nature. Supply intercostal muscles and skin.
- Intercostal arteries:
  - Posterior intercostal arteries (branch of costocervical trunk and thoracic aorta).
  - Anterior intercostal arteries (branch of internal thoracic and musculophrenic artery).

- Intercostal veins:
  - On right side
    - 1st drain into superior vena cava
    - 2nd–11th drain into azygos vein.
  - On left side
    - 1st drain into left brachiocephalic trunk
    - 2nd–4th drain into left superior intercostal vein
    - 5th–8th drain into accessory hemiazygos vein
    - 9th–11th drain into hemiazygos vein.

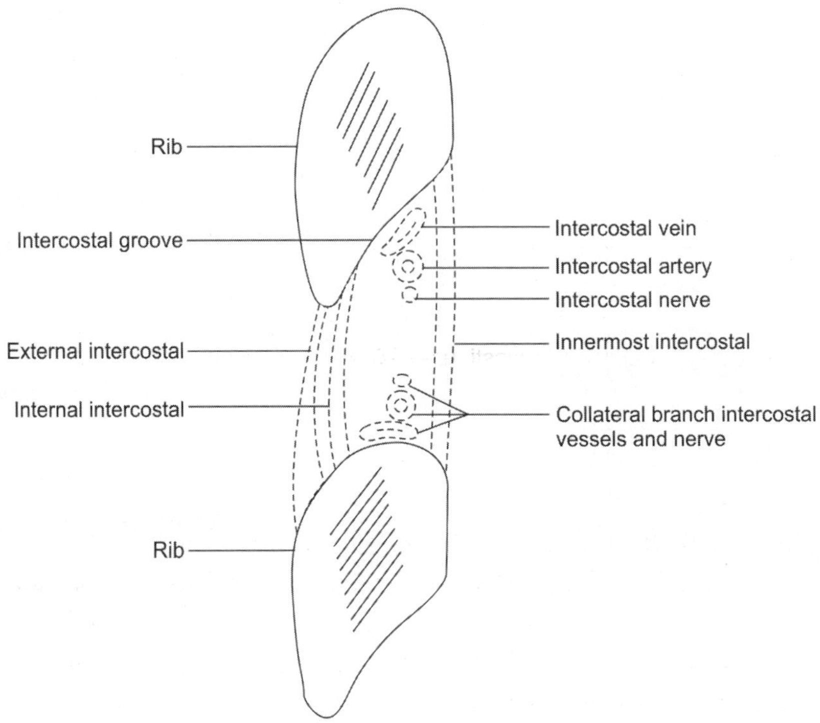

Figure 5.2: Intercostal space—parasagittal section (*For color version, see Plate 9*)

KEY FEATURES

- The neurovascular bundle of each intercostal space lies in the intercostal groove which lies in the lower part of the rib above
- Each intercostal artery and nerve gives a collateral branch which runs along the upper border of the rib below
- Therefore, the safe area is the center of the intercostal space.

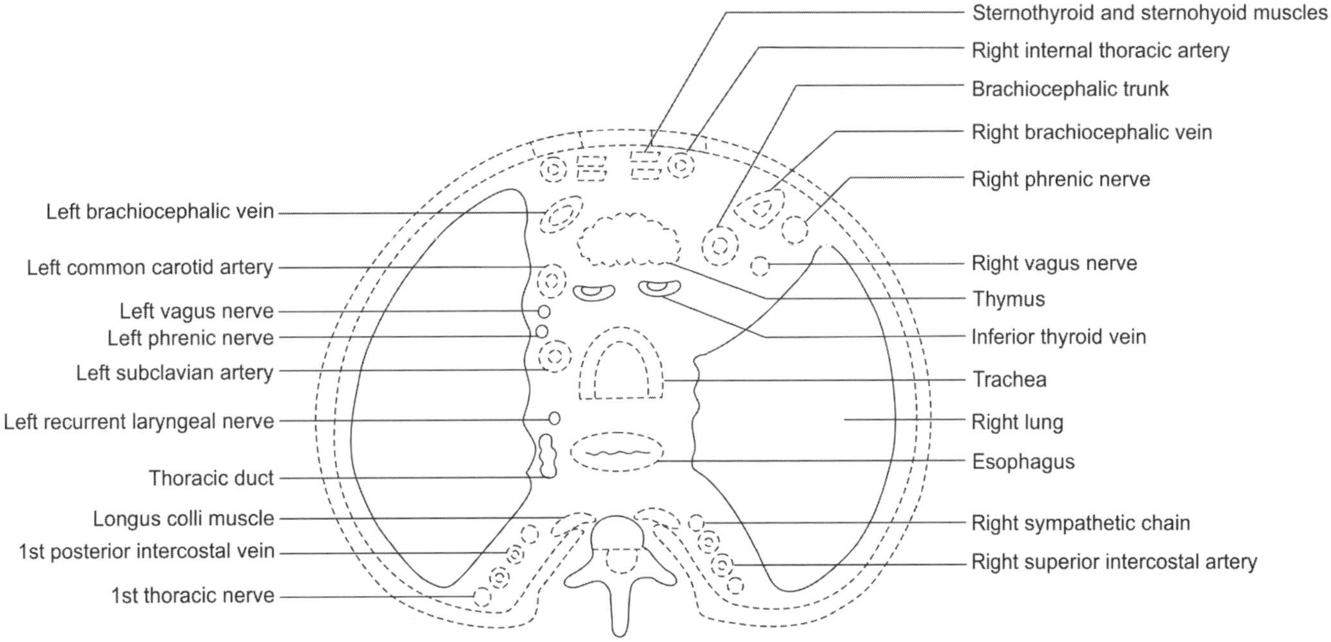

Figure 5.3: Superior mediastinum—TS (*For color version, see Plate 10*)

KEY FEATURES

- It is an area which lies behind manubrium sterni, in front of upper thoracic vertebrae and between two lungs above bifurcation of trachea
- All large veins (superior vena cava, right and left brachiocephalic veins) are on right side
- All large arteries (brachiocephalic trunk, left common carotid and left subclavian) are on left side
- There is sufficient dead space on right side for veins to expand thus tumors of mediastinum project to right side.

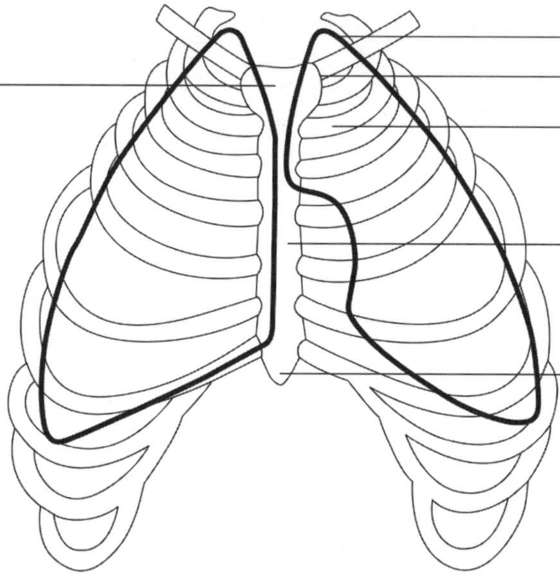

Figure 5.4: Pleural reflections (*For color version, see Plate 10*)

KEY FEATURES

- Since rib inclines at an angle, the apex of lung projects into neck
- Cervical pleura: a point one inch above the junction of middle 1/3rd and medial 1/3rd of clavicle to the sterno-clavicular joint
- Costal pleura: On both sides it starts from sternoclavicular joint to sternal angle. On right side it descends vertically to xiphisternal joint. On left side it descends vertically till 4th costal cartilage and then turns left to reach 6th costal cartilage 3 cm from midline.
- Costodiaphragmatic pleura:
  - On right side from xiphisternal joint to 8th rib.
  - On left side from 6th costal cartilage to 8th rib in midclavicular line, then crosses 10th rib in midaxillary line to reach 12th rib 2 cm lateral to spine of 12th thoracic vertebra.
- Inferior margin lung lies along 6th, 8th and 10th ribs
- Inferior margin of pleura lies along 8th, 10th and 12th ribs.

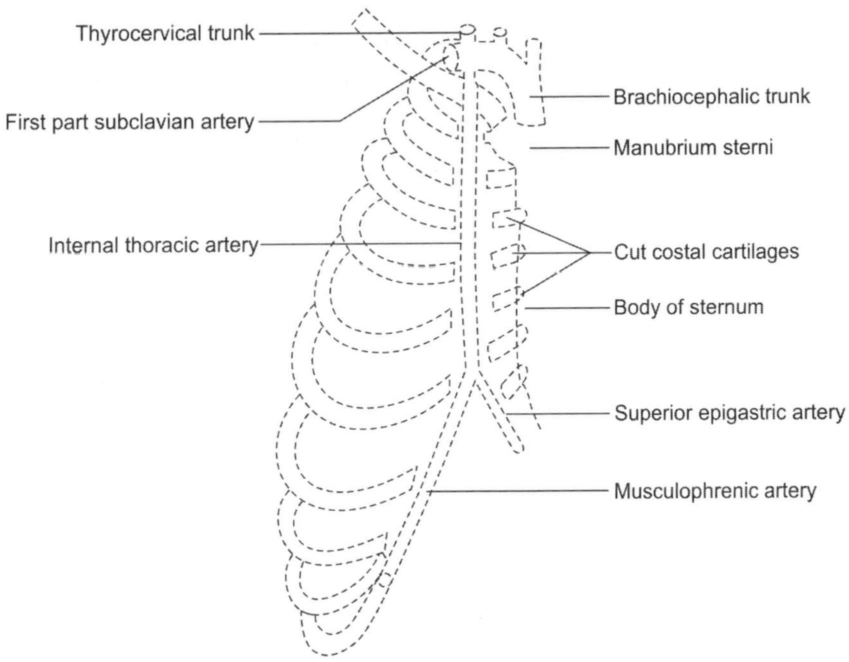

Figure 5.5: Internal thoracic artery

KEY FEATURES

- Arises from first part subclavian artery lower surface opposite thyrocervical trunk
- Descends behind clavicle and upper six costal cartilages 1 cm lateral to sternum where it divides into superior epigastric and musculophrenic arteries
- Superior epigastric enters rectus sheath and musculophrenic gives anterior intercostal branches to 7th and 8th intercostal spaces. It ends by supplying diaphragm and anterior abdominal wall.

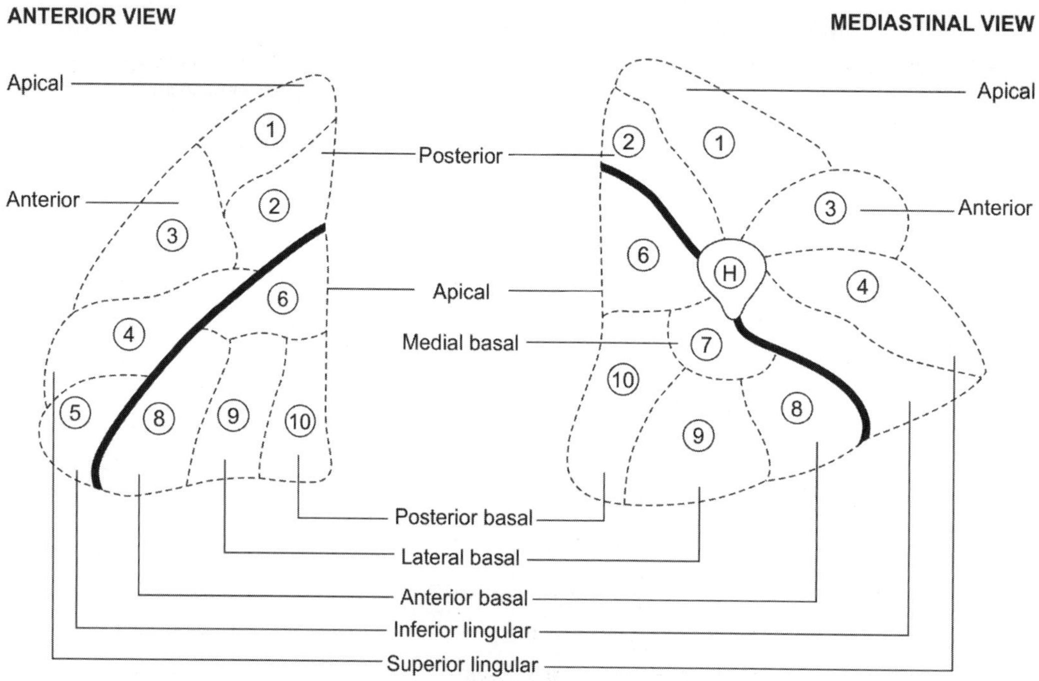

Figure 5.6: Bronchopulmonary segments of left lung—anterior and mediastinal view

KEY FEATURES

- Bronchopulmonary segment is a well-defined wedge-shaped sector of lung
- It is an anatomical, functional and surgical unit of lung
- Apex of the segment lies towards the hilum of lung and base towards surface
- Each segment has its own artery, nerve supply and lymphatic drainage but the veins are intersegmental.

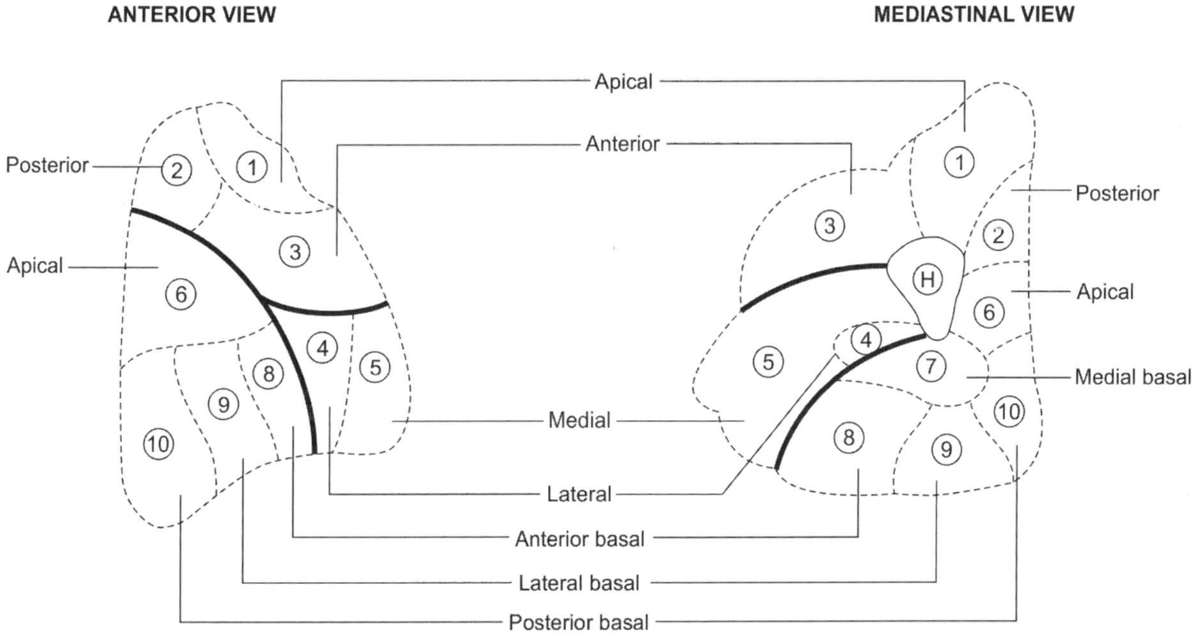

Figure 5.7: Bronchopulmonary segments of right lung—anterior and mediastinal view

KEY FEATURES

- Clinically the knowledge of the bronchopulmonary segments allows the surgeon to do segmental resection of lung
- It is nature's defense mechanism to localize certain chronic diseases like tuberculosis, benign neoplasm, bronchiectasis, etc.

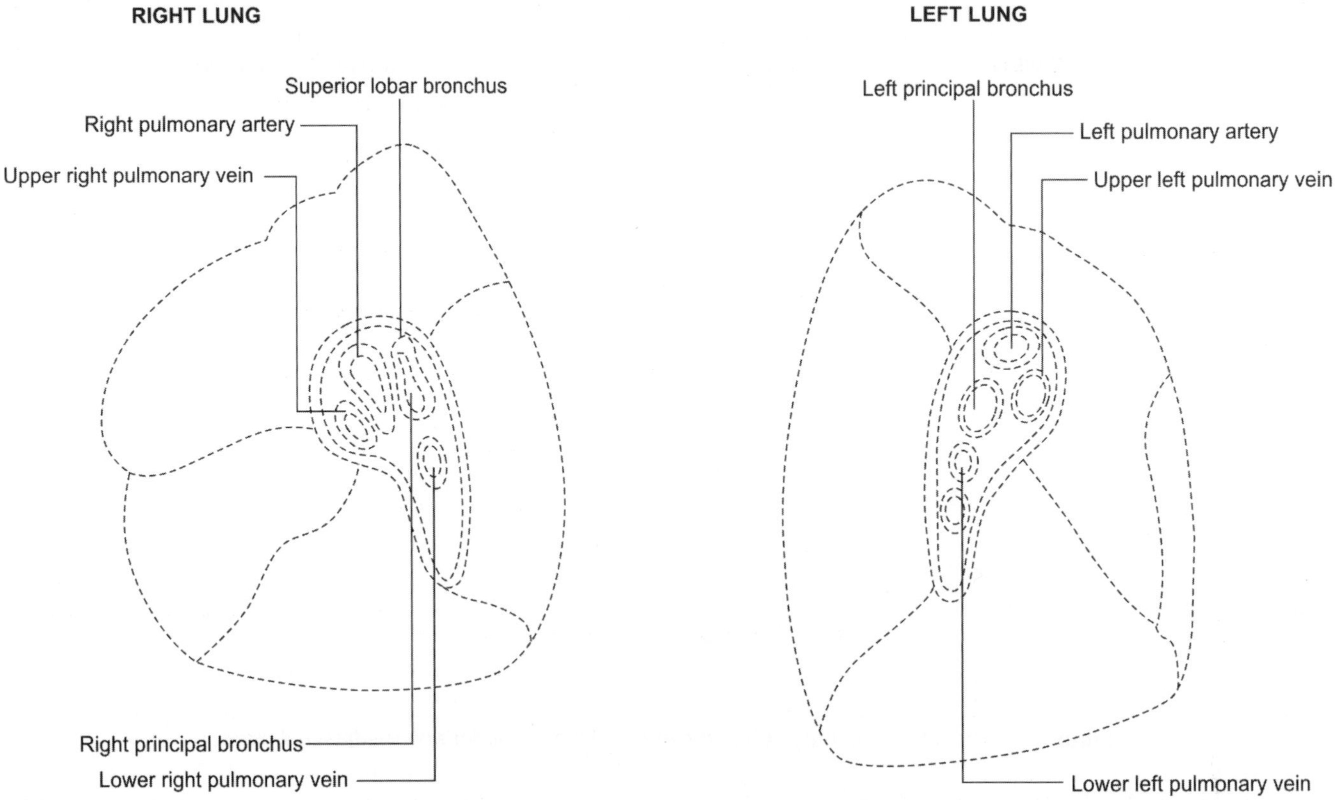

Figure 5.8: Hilum of lungs—right and left lung

KEY FEATURES

- Hilum is an area on the mediastinal surface of lung through which structures enter or leave the lung
- Root of the lung is a broad, short pedicle connecting medial surface of lung with mediastinum. It consists of structures entering or leaving the lung. It lies opposite T5–T7 vertebrae.

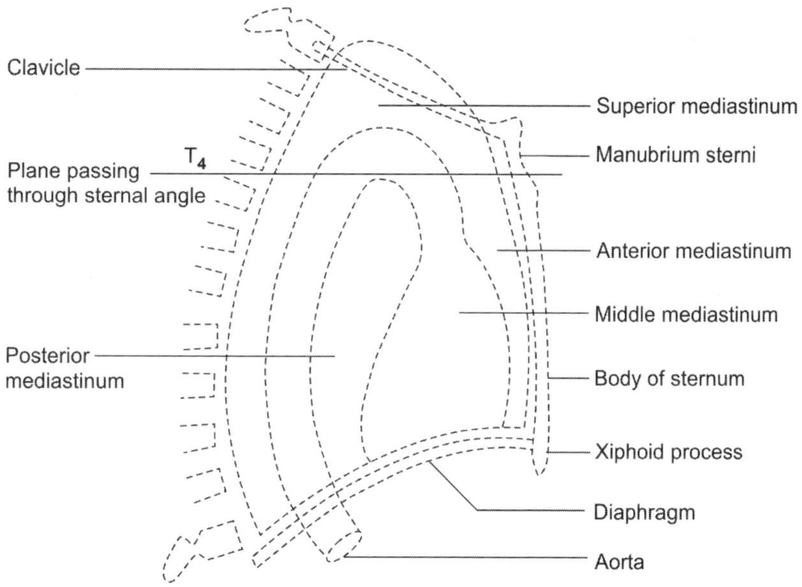

Figure 5.9: Subdivisions of mediastinum

KEY FEATURES

- Mediastinum is divided into superior and inferior components by transthoracic plane passing sternal angle anteriorly and T4 vertebra posteriorly
- The superior mediastinum contains great vessels of thorax, nerves and trachea
- Inferior mediastinum is divided into anterior, middle and posterior components
- The middle mediastinum contains heart enclosed in pericardium
- The posterior mediastinum contains descending aorta, esophagus, thoracic duct and vagus nerves.

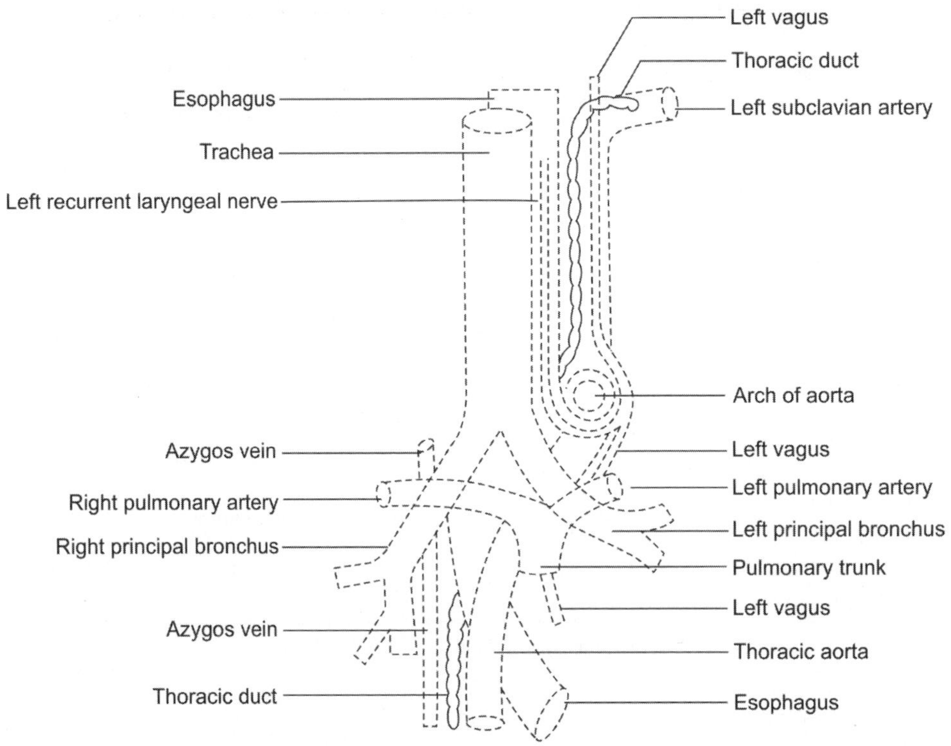

Figure 5.10: Left recurrent laryngeal nerve

KEY FEATURES

- The left vagus as it enters thorax descends anterolateral to the arch of aorta
- Just posterior to ligamentum arteriosum it gives off recurrent laryngeal nerve
- The recurrent laryngeal nerve winds around the arch of aorta to reach it's posteromedial aspect
- Then, the nerve ascends upward in the interval between trachea and esophagus alongwith thoracic duct to enter neck.

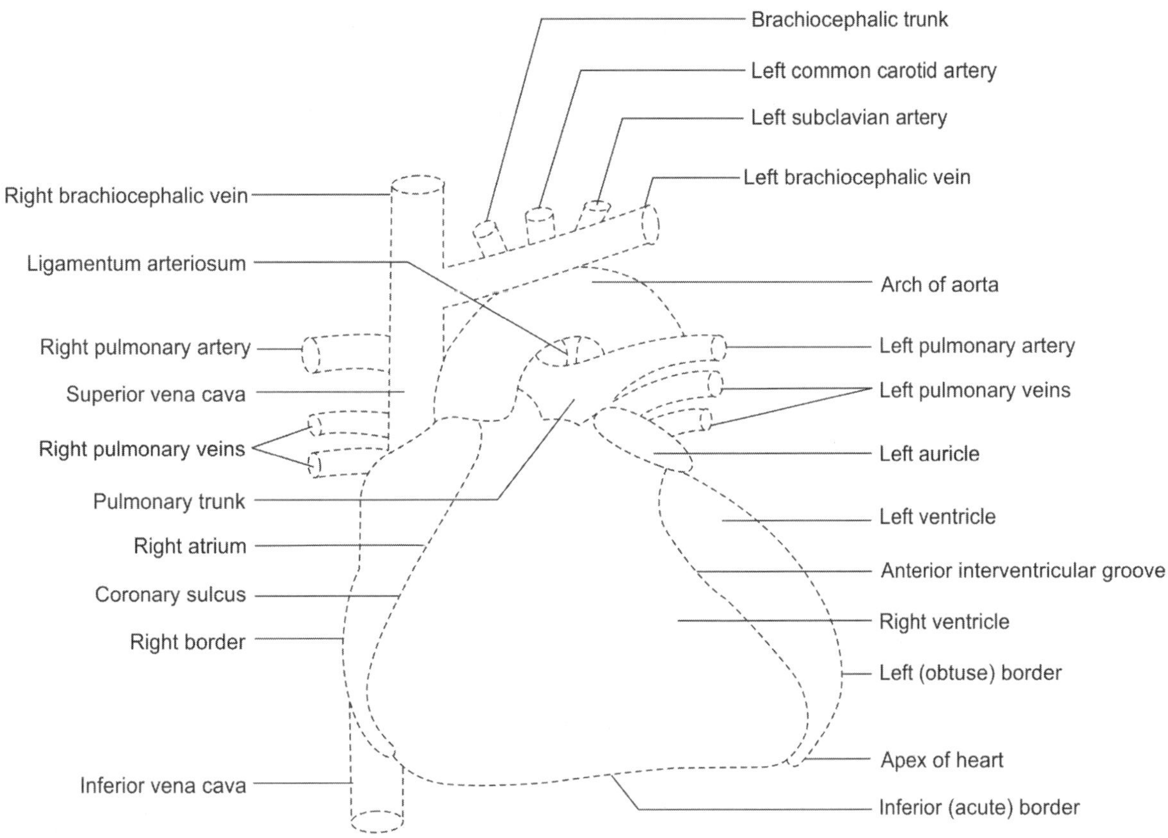

Figure 5.11: Heart and great vessels—anterior view

KEY FEATURES

- The anterior aspect of heart is the sternocostal surface
- From right to left it is formed by right atrium, anterior part coronary sulcus, right ventricle anterior part interventricular groove and part of left ventricle
- The right ventricle makes up most of the sternocostal surface
- Right coronary artery runs in the coronary sulcus, whereas anterior interventricular ramus a branch of left coronary artery runs in interventricular groove.

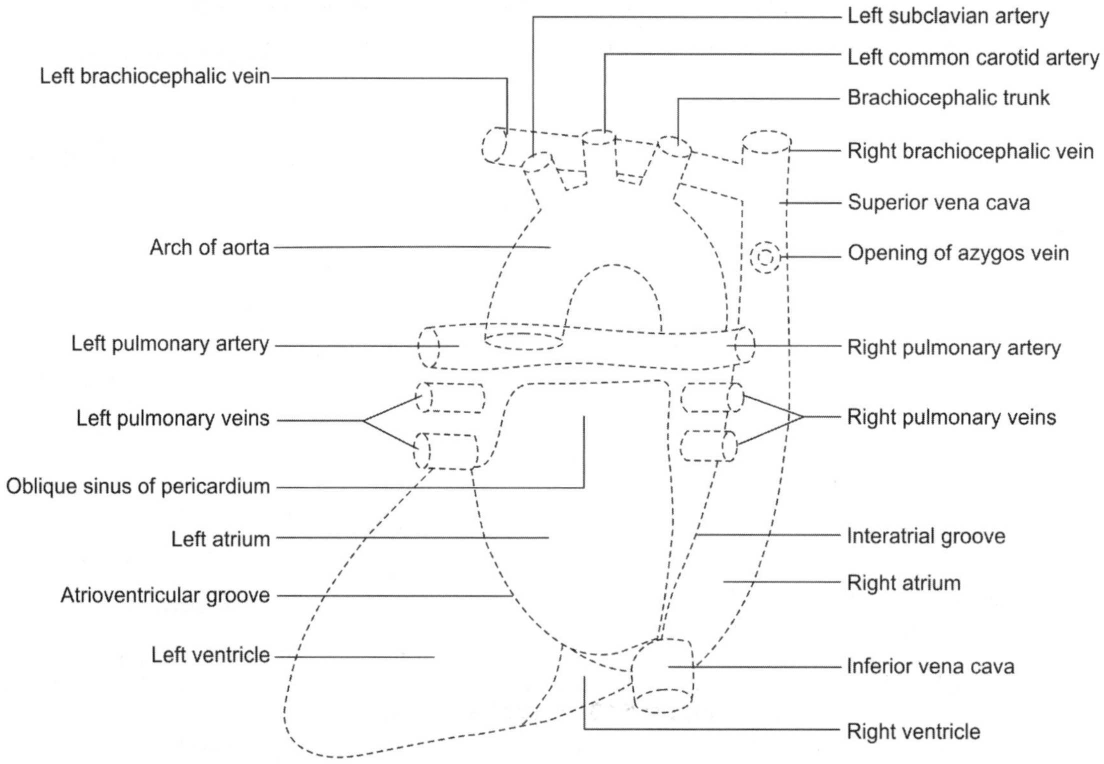

Figure 5.12: Heart and great vessels—posterior view

KEY FEATURES

- Base of the heart faces backwards and to the right
- The left atrium forms 2/3rd of the base and the rest is formed by right atrium
- Four pulmonary veins open into left atrium whereas superior and inferior vena cava open into right atrium
- Inter atrial groove separates right and left atrium.

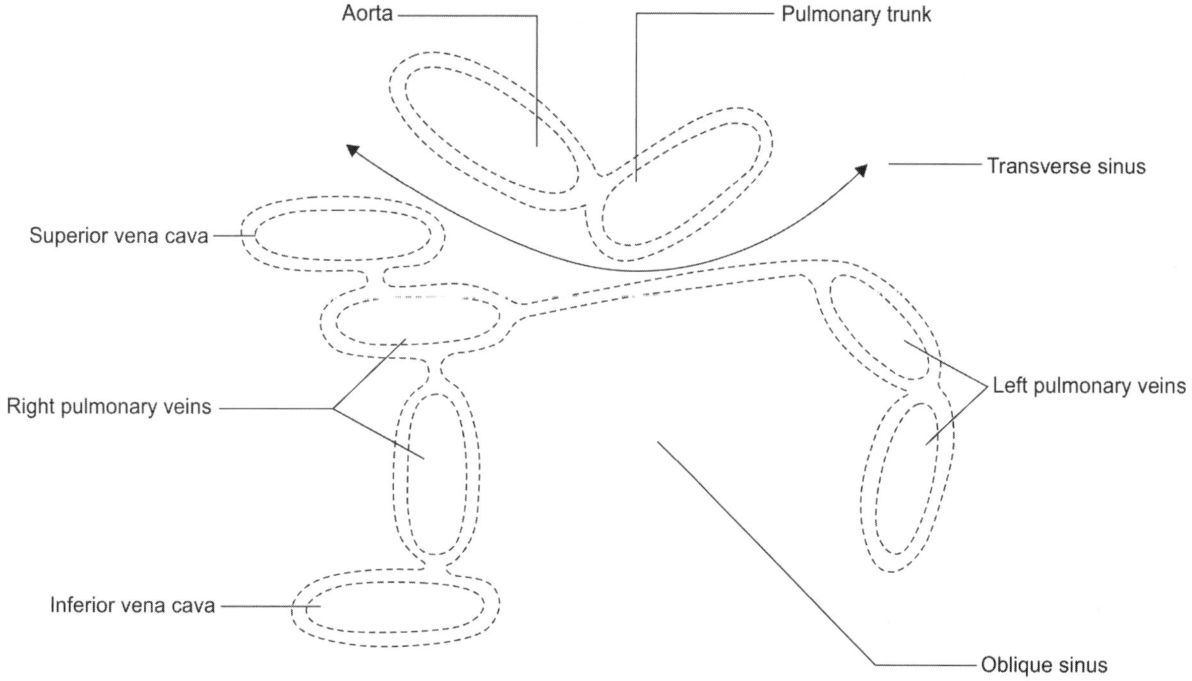

Figure 5.13: Pericardial sinuses

KEY FEATURES

- Transverse sinus—lies between arterial and venous ends of heart
  - Bounded anteriorly by ascending aorta and pulmonary trunk
  - Posteriorly by superior vena cava and superior pulmonary veins.
- Oblique sinus is a recess of serous pericardium, lies behind left atrium and is "J" shaped
  - Bounded on the right by right pulmonary veins and inferior vena cava
  - On left by left pulmonary veins
- Cause—absorption of four pulmonary veins into left atrium
- Function—allows distension of left atrium.

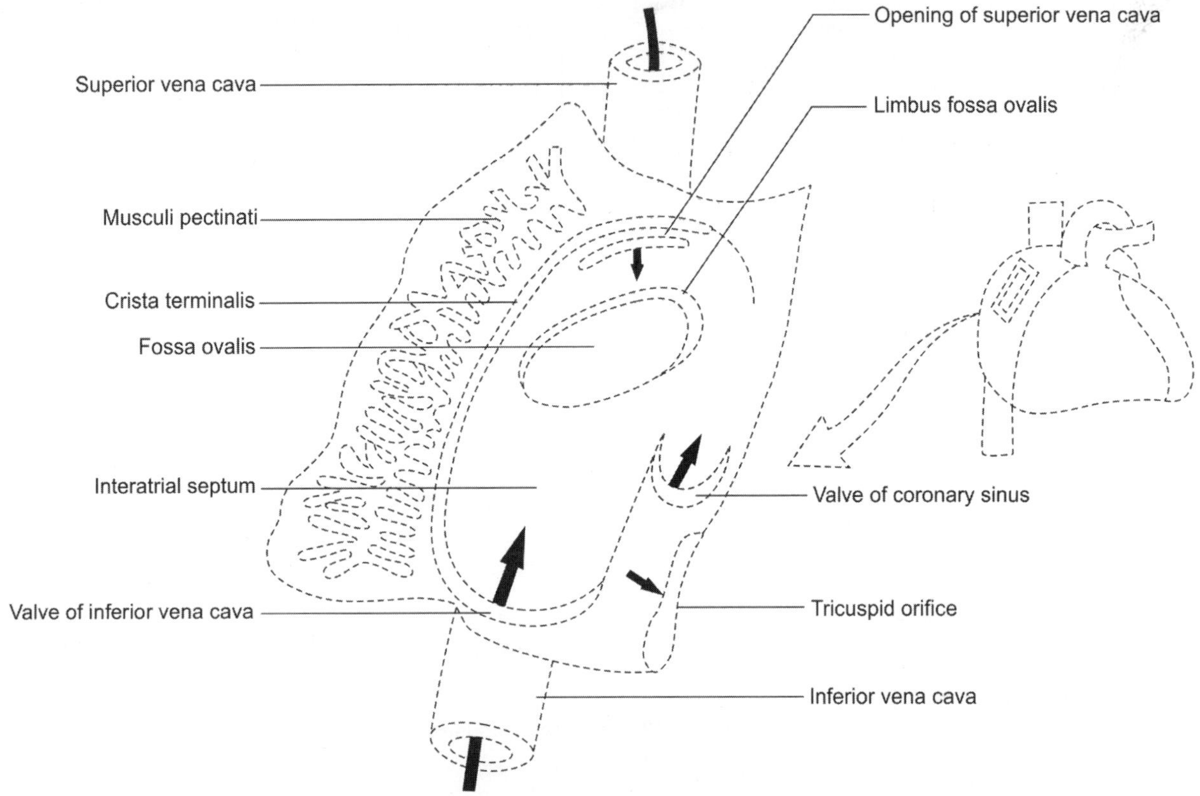

Figure 5.14: Interior of right atrium

KEY FEATURES

- It has a rough part which represents primitive atrium. It is separated from smooth part by crista terminalis. All veins open in smooth part
- Two atria are separated by a septum. The septum has limbus fossa ovalis which represents free margin of septum secundum and fossa ovalis which represents septum primum
- Following veins open into right atrium superior vena cava, inferior vena cava, coronary sinus, Thebesian veins and right atrioventricular orifice.

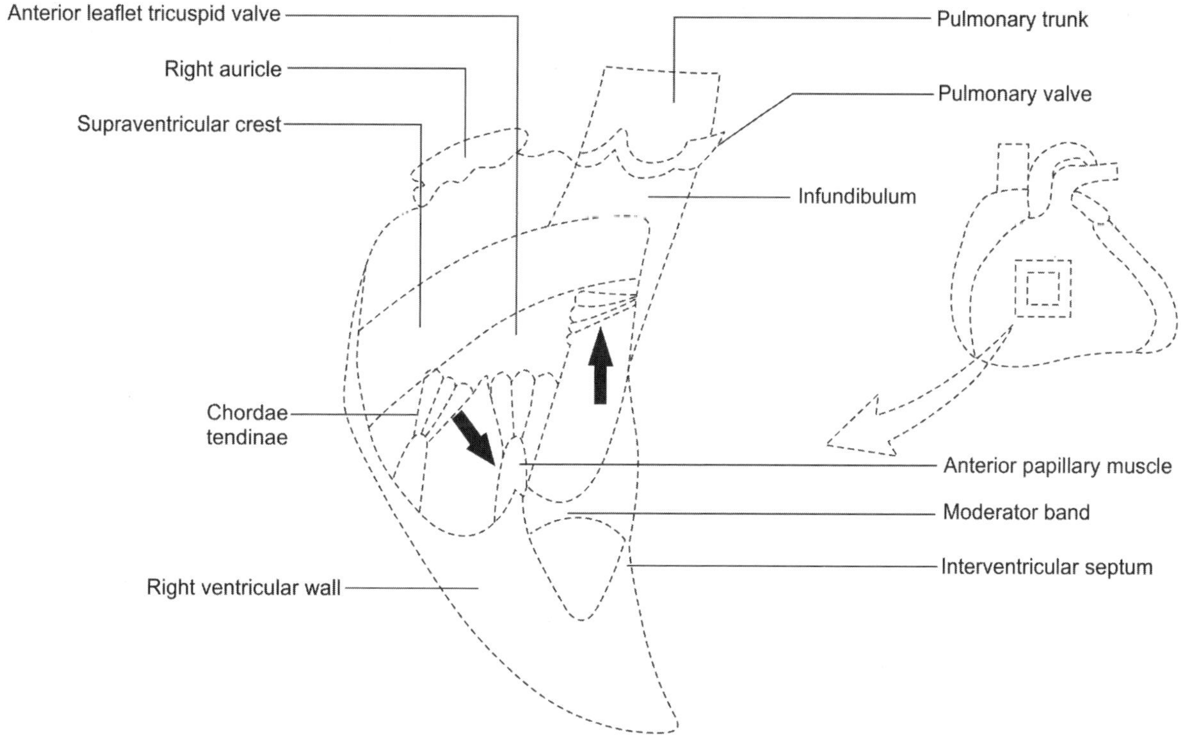

Figure 5.15: Interior of right ventricle

KEY FEATURES

It has two parts—inflow and outflow tract.

i. Inflow tract represents primitive ventricle. It is large and lies below supraventricular crest. It has trabeculae carnii. There are three papillary muscles, anterior, posterior and septal. There is a moderator band between septum and anterior papillary muscle. It conveys right bundle branch. The function of moderator band is to prevent ventricular over distension.

ii. Outflow tract is very smooth and lies above supraventricular crest. It ends at pulmonary valves.

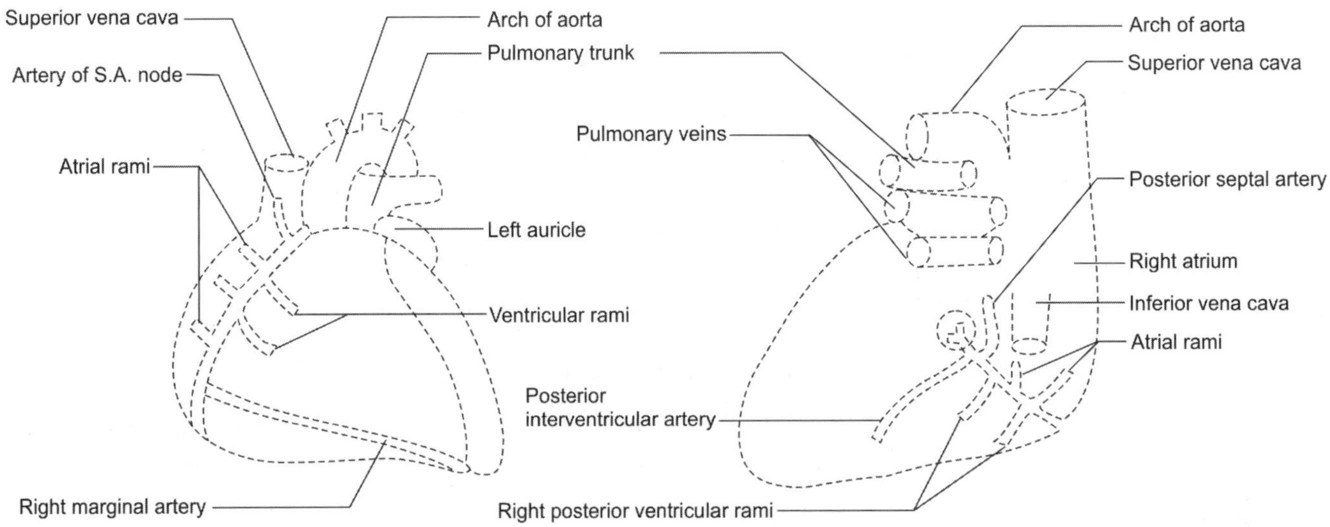

Figure 5.16: Right coronary artery—anterior and posterior view

KEY FEATURES

- Origin—anterior aortic sinus
- Course—on the sternocostal surface runs down in right atrioventricular (AV) groove (right anterior coronary sulcus)
- Then runs on the diaphragmatic surface in posterior atrioventricular (AV) groove (right posterior coronary sulcus to reach posterior interventricular groove
- Branches:
  - Atrial
  - Anterior ventricular ramifications, one large ramus is called marginal artery
  - Posterior ventricular branch
  - Posterior septal artery.
  - Posterior interventricular artery that runs up to the apex and supplies both ventricles and AV node.

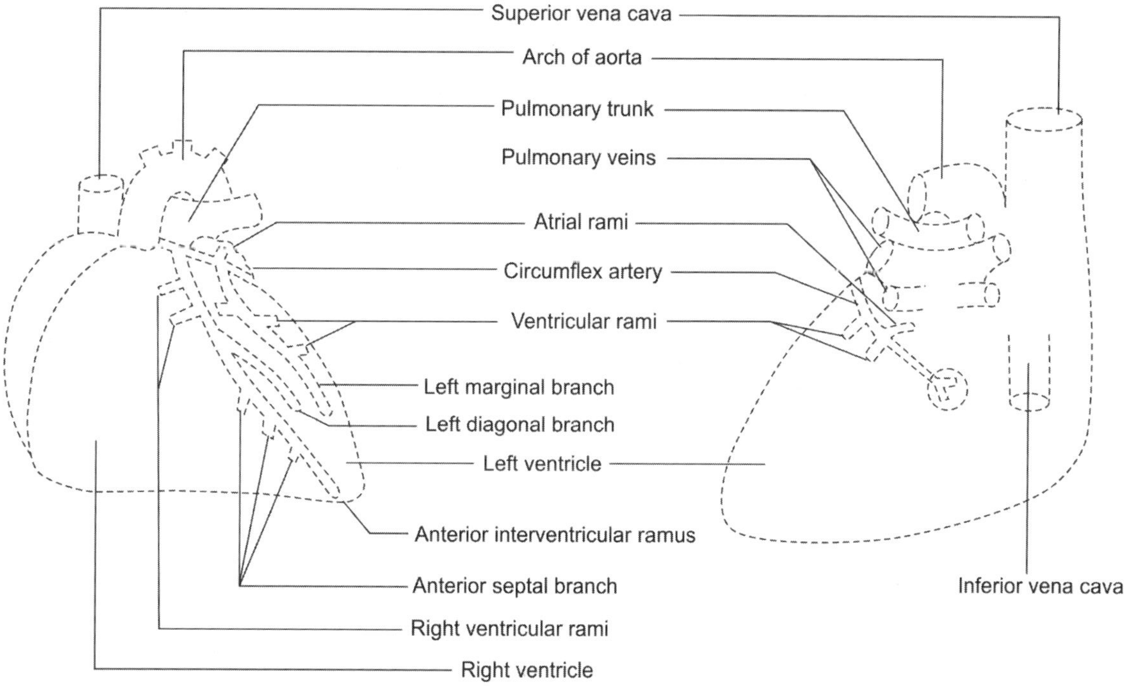

Figure 5.17: Left coronary artery—anterior and posterior view

KEY FEATURES

- It arises from left posterior aortic sinus
- Runs between arch of aorta and pulmonary trunk. It divides into two branches:
  i. Anterior interventricular which runs towards apex and anastomosis with posterior interventricular artery. It supplies anterior part interventricular septum, left bundle branch and both ventricles.
  ii. Circumflex artery which winds around the left margin of heart. It runs in left posterior coronary sulcus and anastomoses with right coronary artery.
  Its main branch is left marginal artery. The circumflex artery supplies left atrium and ventricle. Left diagonal branch is variable.

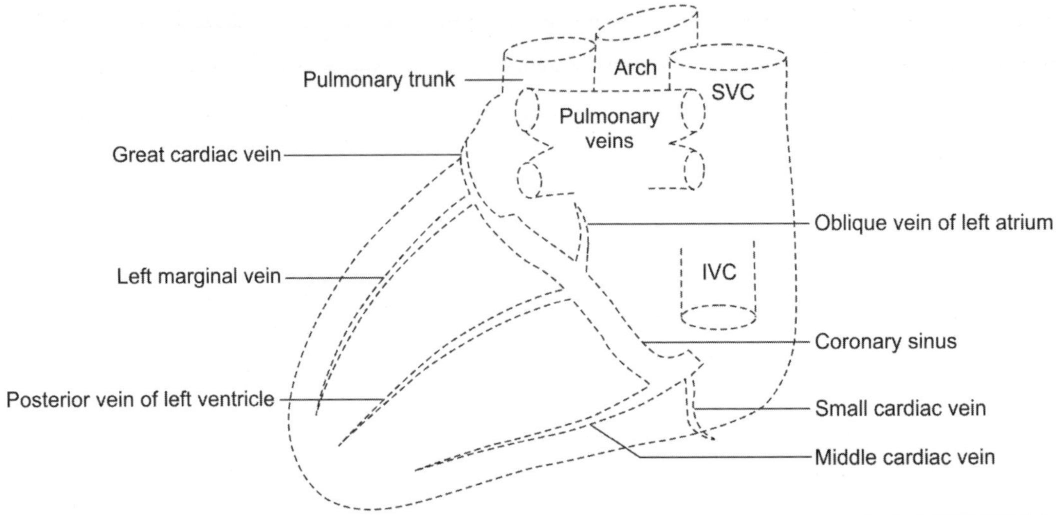

Figure 5.18: Venous drainage of heart—posterior view

KEY FEATURES

The veins which drain the heart are:

- Coronary sinus which lies in left posterior coronary sulcus. Its tributaries are:
  - Great cardiac vein
  - Middle cardiac vein
  - Small cardiac vein
  - Posterior vein of left ventricle
  - Oblique vein of left atrium (vein of Marshall)
- Anterior cardiac veins
- Venae cordis minimae (Thebesian veins).

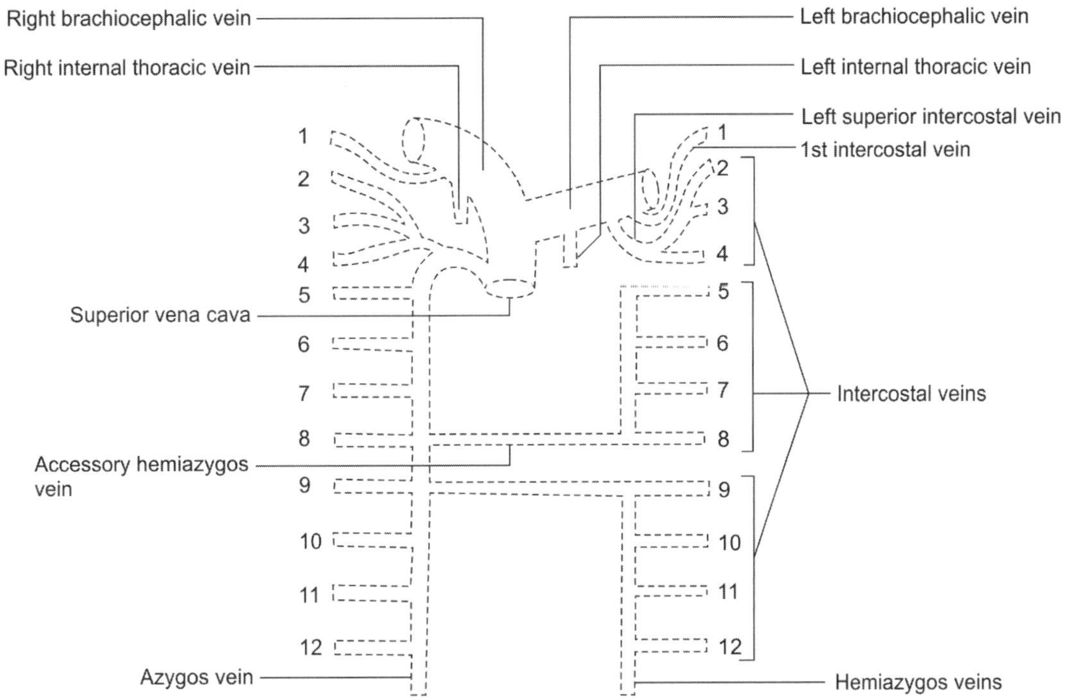

Figure 5.19: Azygos system of veins

KEY FEATURES

- It drains thoracic cage and upper lumbar region. It is present only on right side
- Connects superior and inferior vena cava and has valves
- Formed by the union of right subcostal and right ascending lumbar veins at T12 vertebra
- It ends at the level of T4 by arching over the right bronchus and opens in superior vena cava
- On right side, 1st posterior intercostal vein opens into right brachiocephalic vein and rest in azygos vein
- On left side, 1st–4th posterior intercostal veins open into left brachiocephalic vein, 5th–8th unite to form accessory hemiazygos which opens in azygos and 9th–12th unite to form hemiazygos which opens in azygos.

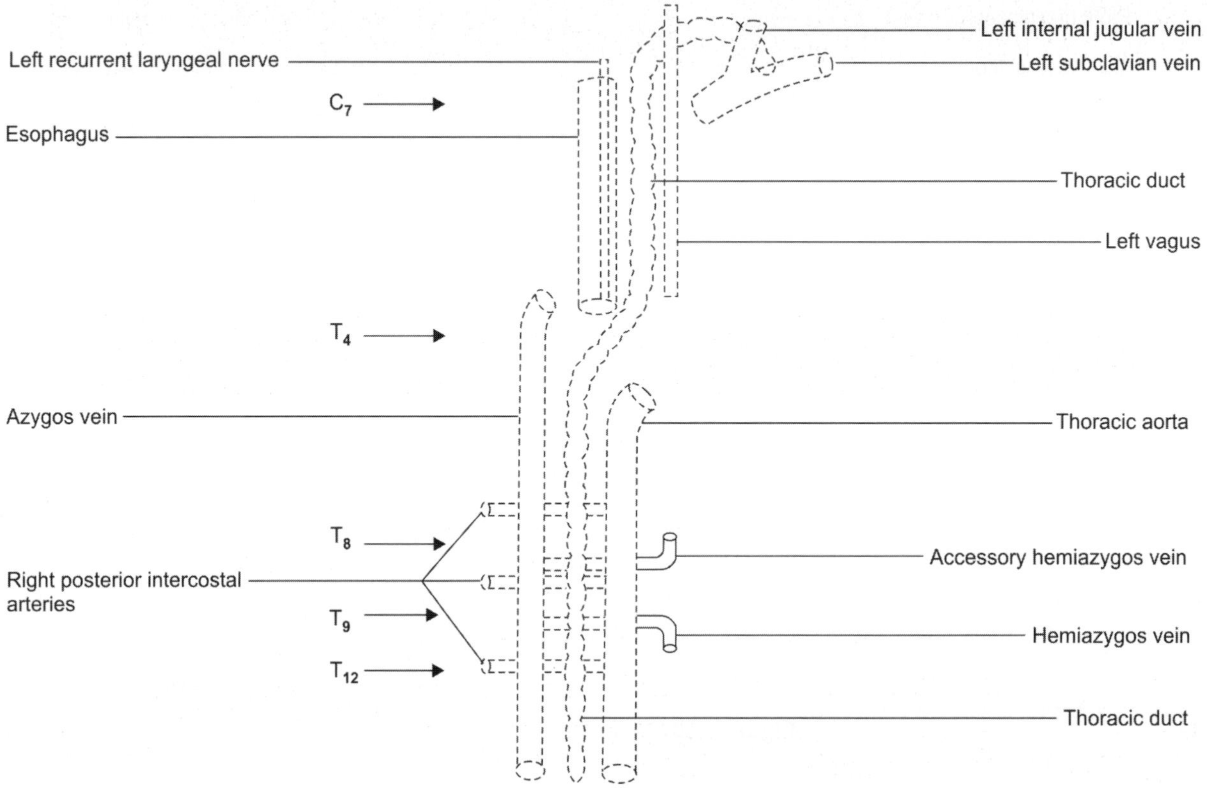

Figure 5.20: Thoracic duct

KEY FEATURES

- Largest lymphatic trunk in the body, appears beaded due to many valves
- Drains entire body except right side head and neck, right side chest, right lung, right side heart and right surface of liver
- Extent—from lower border of T12 (cisterna chyli) to the junction of left internal jugular vein and left subclavian vein
- Length 45 cm, enters thorax through aortic opening
- In lower half runs on right side in posterior mediastinum, at T4–5 crosses to the left and enters superior mediastinum
- It then enters neck, arches at C7, 3–4 cm above clavicle and ends at the junction of left internal jugular vein and left subclavian vein.

CHAPTER 6

Abdomen and Pelvis

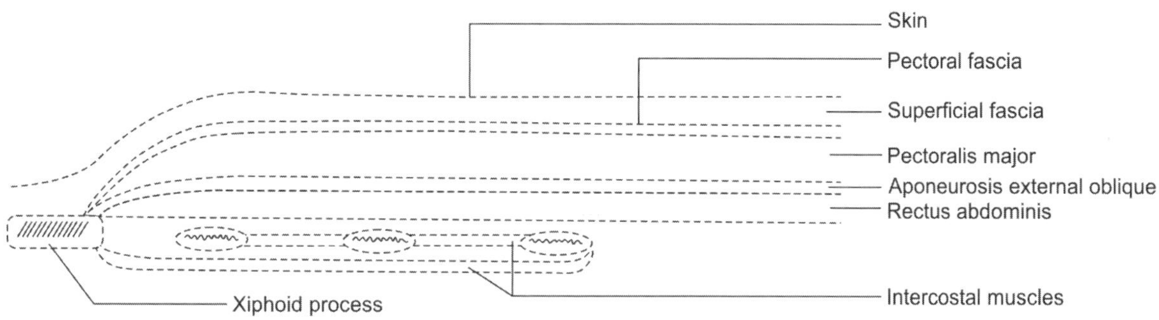

Figure 6.1: Rectus sheath transverse section—above costal margin (*For color version, see Plate 11*)

KEY FEATURES

- Anterior wall—external oblique aponeurosis
- Posterior wall—formed by 5–7th costal cartilages.

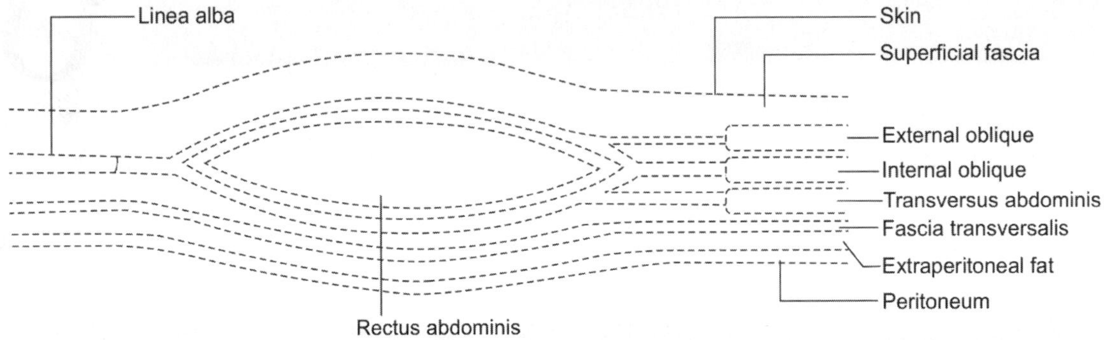

Figure 6.2: Rectus sheath transverse section—between costal margin and anterior superior iliac spine
(*For color version, see Plate 11*)

KEY FEATURES

- Anterior wall—formed by the fusion of external oblique aponeurosis and anterior lamina of internal oblique aponeurosis
- Posterior wall—formed by the fusion of posterior lamina of internal oblique aponeurosis and transversus abdominis muscle.

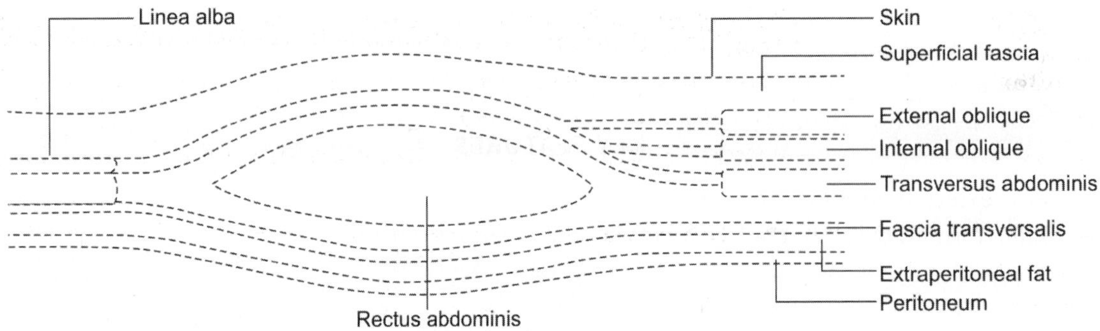

Figure 6.3: Rectus sheath transverse section—between anterior superior iliac spine and pubic symphysis
(*For color version, see Plate 11*)

KEY FEATURES

- Anterior wall—formed by the fusion of external oblique, internal oblique aponeurosis and transversus abdominis muscle
- Posterior wall—it is deficient and presents a free margin of all the three muscles called arcuate line.

There are three intertendinous junctions which fuse with rectus sheath thereby increasing the efficiency of the muscle.

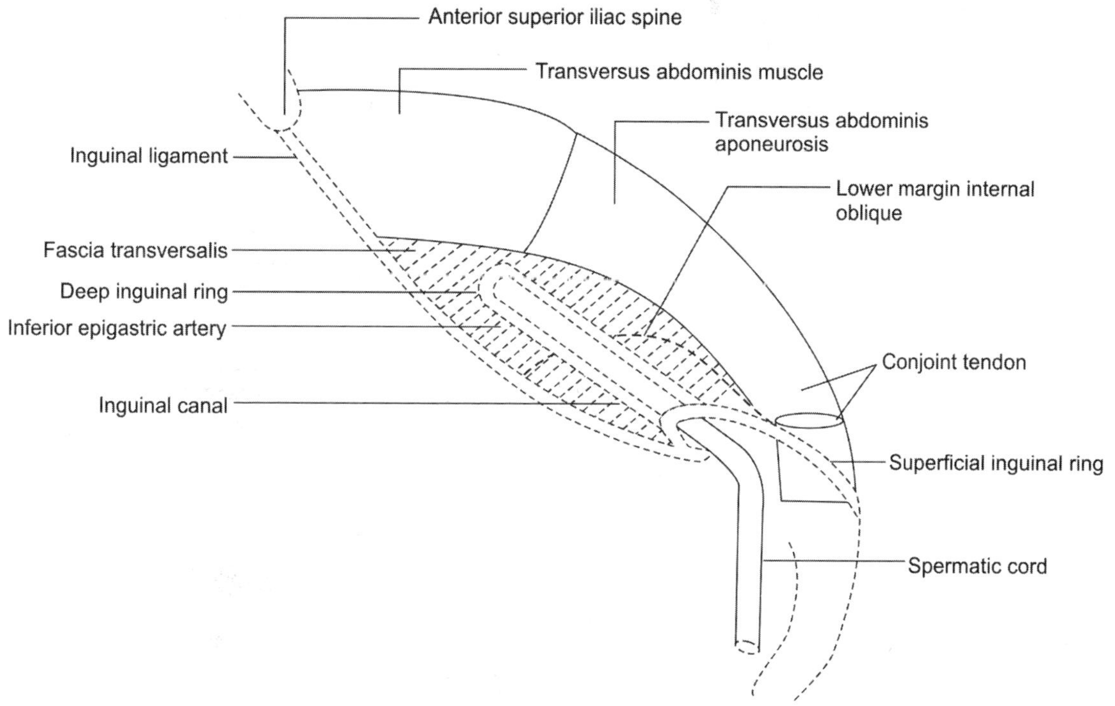

Figure 6.4: Inguinal canal (*For color version, see Plate 12*)

KEY FEATURES

- Oblique intramuscular passage, lies over medial half inguinal ligament, it is 4 cm long, running between deep and superficial inguinal rings
- Anterior wall—skin, superficial fascia, external oblique muscle. It is reinforced by internal oblique muscle in lateral 1/3rd
- Posterior wall—fascia transversalis. Conjoint tendon in medial 1/3rd. Reflected part inguinal ligament in medial most part
- Floor—inguinal ligament and abdominal part lacunar ligament
- Roof—lower arched fibers of internal oblique and transversus abdominis muscle.

  It contains ilioinguinal nerve and spermatic cord in males/round ligament in females.

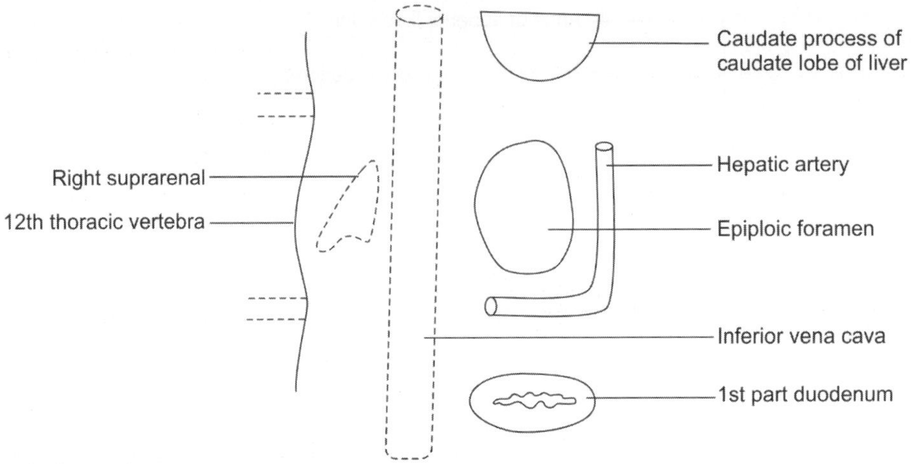

Figure 6.5: Epiploic foramen (*For color version, see Plate 12*)

KEY FEATURES

- A vertical slit through which lesser sac continues with greater sac
- Location—behind right free margin of lesser omentum
- Boundaries:
  - Anterior—right free margin of lesser omentum and vertical part hepatic artery
  - Posterior—inferior vena cava and right suprarenal gland
  - Superior—caudate process of caudate lobe of liver
  - Inferior—first part of duodenum and transverse part of hepatic artery.

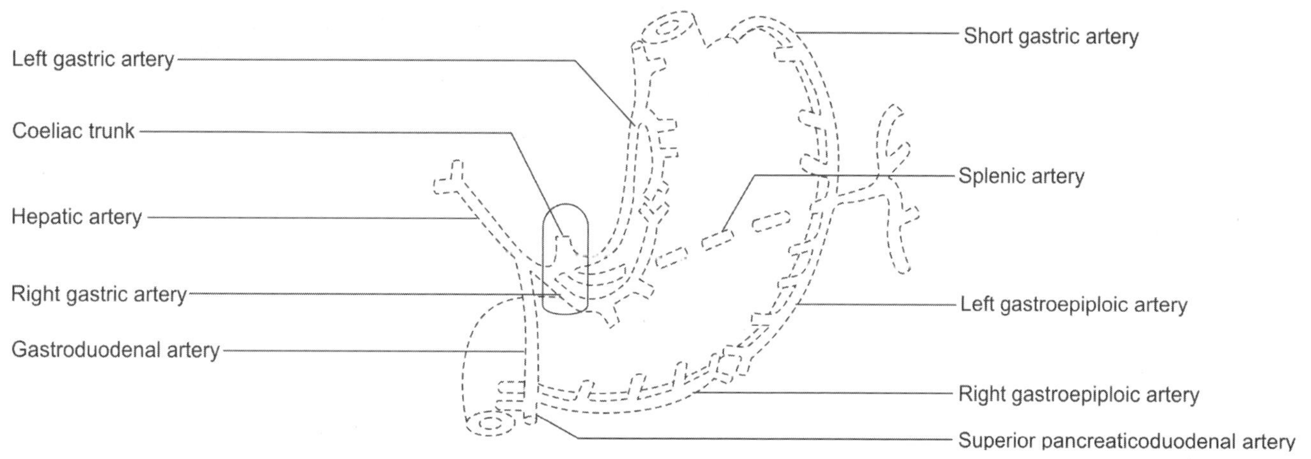

Figure 6.6: Blood supply—stomach

KEY FEATURES

- It is supplied by branches of coeliac trunk (foregut)
- Vessels along lesser curvature:
  - Left gastric—direct branch of coeliac trunk
  - Right gastric—branch of common hepatic artery.
- Vessels along greater curvature:
  - Short gastric—branch of splenic artery
  - Left gastroepiploic—branch of splenic artery
  - Right gastroepiploic—branch of gastroduodenal artery.

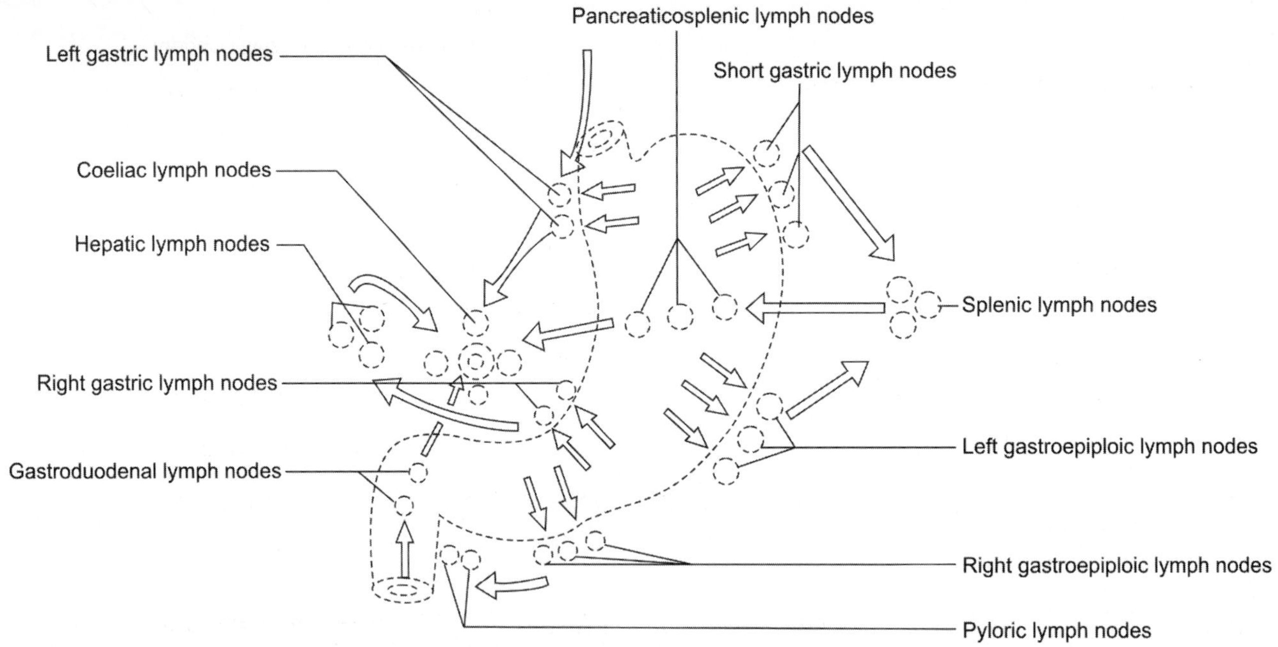

Figure 6.7: Lymphatic drainage—stomach

KEY FEATURES

- The lymph nodes are arranged along the arteries which supply stomach
- They drain approximately the same areas as supplied by the arteries
- The lymph nodes can be arranged in following groups:
  - Along lesser curvature: Left gastric lymph node
  - Pyloric antrum and canal along lesser curvature: Right gastric lymph node
  - Along fundus: Short gastric lymph node
  - Along greater curvature: Left gastroepiploic lymph node
  - Pyloric antrum and canal along greater curvature: Right gastroepiploic lymph node
  - Along splenic artery: Pancreaticosplenic lymph node.

  All the lymph nodes drain directly into coeliac lymph node or indirectly via splenic and hepatic lymph node.

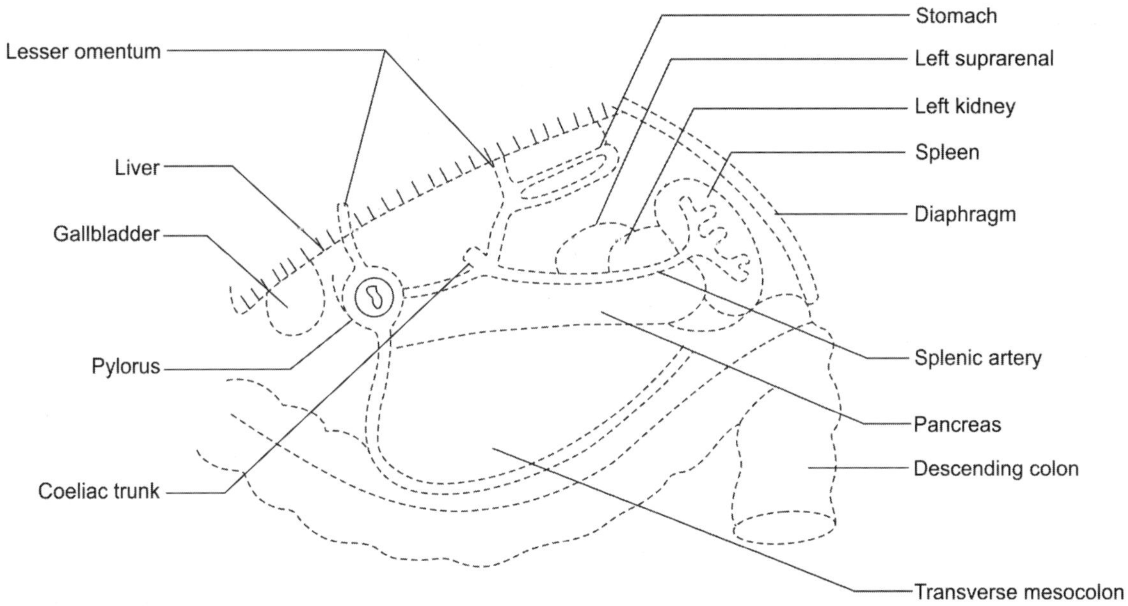

Figure 6.8: Structures in stomach bed

KEY FEATURES

- The structures along posterior abdominal wall which are related to stomach constitute stomach bed. Lesser sac (omental bursa) intervenes between stomach and posterior abdominal wall
- These structures are:
  - Transverse mesocolon
  - Pancreas
  - Splenic artery
  - Diaphragm
  - Left suprarenal
  - Left kidney
  - Spleen
  - Left colic flexure.

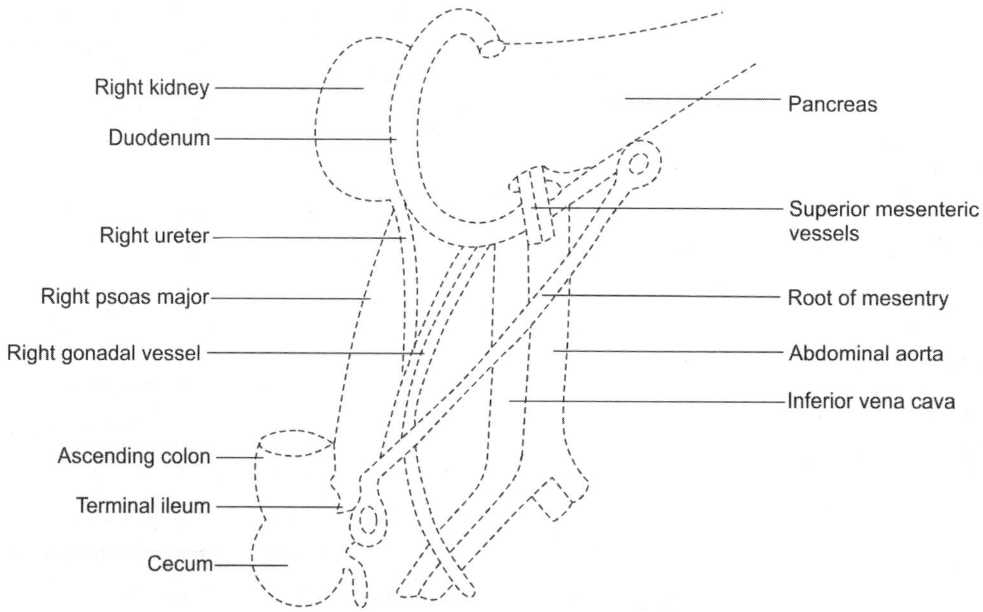

Figure 6.9: Root of mesentery

KEY FEATURES

The attached margin of the peritoneal fold which encloses small intestine is called root of mesentery. It is six inches long.

- Extent: From duodenojejunal flexure (left side L2) to ileocecal junction (upper part right sacroiliac joint)
- It crosses following structures from left to right:
  - 3rd part duodenum
  - Abdominal aorta
  - Inferior vena cava
  - Right gonadal vessels
  - Right ureter
  - Right psoas major.
- Contents:
  - Superior mesenteric arteries and branches
  - Lymphatics
  - Lymph nodes
  - Nerve plexus.

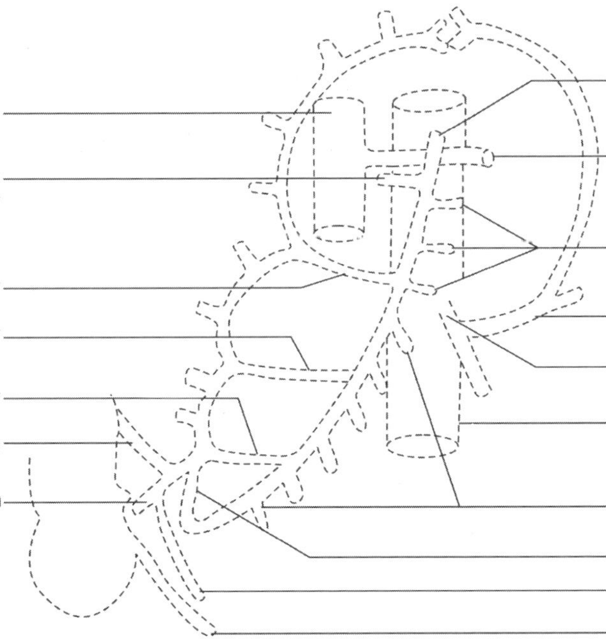

Figure 6.10: Superior mesenteric artery

KEY FEATURES

- Artery of mid gut, arises 1.25 cm below coeliac trunk at the level of L1
- It runs down and towards right, crosses uncinate process and 3rd part of duodenum to enter mesentery
- Branches:
  - From left side—jejunal and ileal branches
  - From right side—
    - Inferior pancreaticoduodenal
    - Middle colic which anastomosis with left colic (branch of inferior mesenteric) at the junction of right 2/3rd and left 1/3rd of transverse colon
    - Right colic
    - Ileocolic. The ileocolic artery gives rise to ileal, colic and cecal branches. Appendicular artery arises from cecal branch.

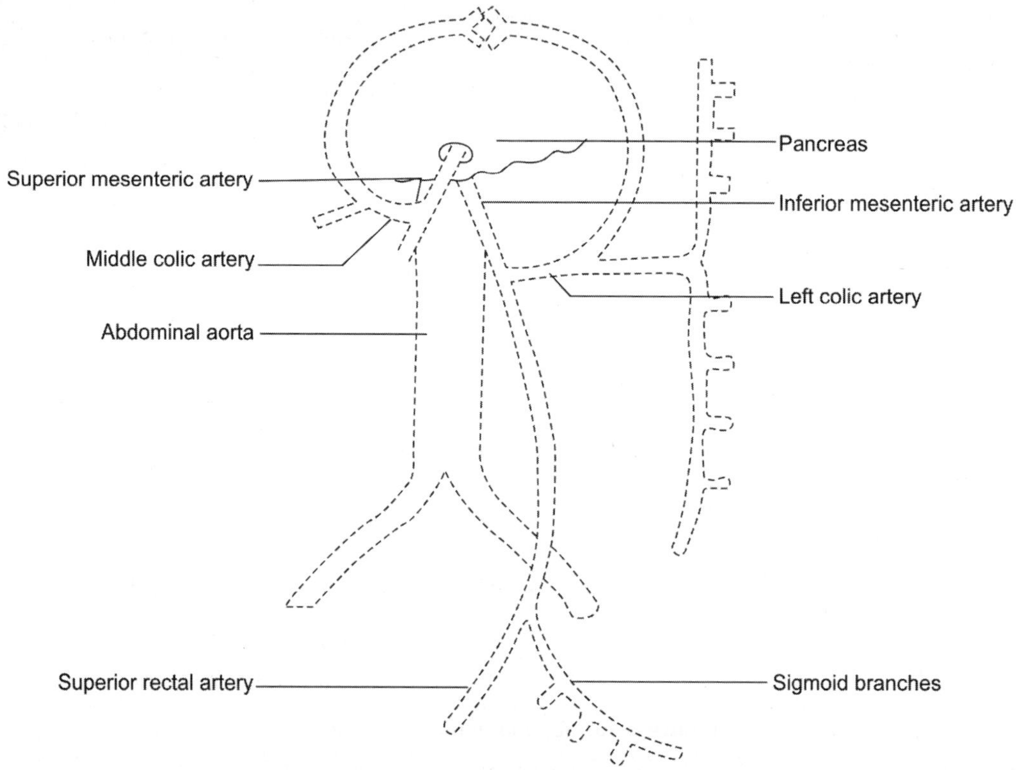

Figure 6.11: Inferior mesenteric artery

KEY FEATURES

- Artery of hind gut, arises 3–4 cm above the bifurcation of aorta, behind 3rd part of duodenum
- It runs downwards and to the left. Crosses the termination of left common iliac artery and continues as superior rectal artery
- Branches:
  - Left colic which anastomosis with middle colic (branch of superior mesenteric) at the junction of right 2/3rd and left 1/3rd of transverse colon
  - Sigmoidal artery.

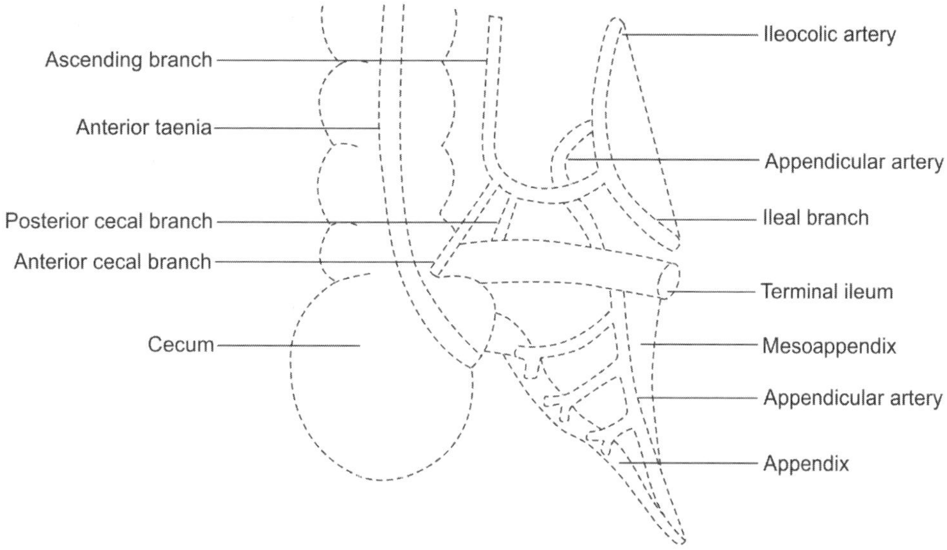

Figure 6.12: Appendix—blood supply

KEY FEATURES

- Appendix arises from posteromedial wall of cecum, 2 cm below ileocecal junction, average size 9 cm
- It has a mesentery called mesoappendix
- It is supplied by appendicular artery which is a branch of ileocolic artery
- The artery enters the mesoappendix to supply the appendix
- Inflammation of appendix causes appendicitis and its pain is referred to umbilicus (T10 dermatome).

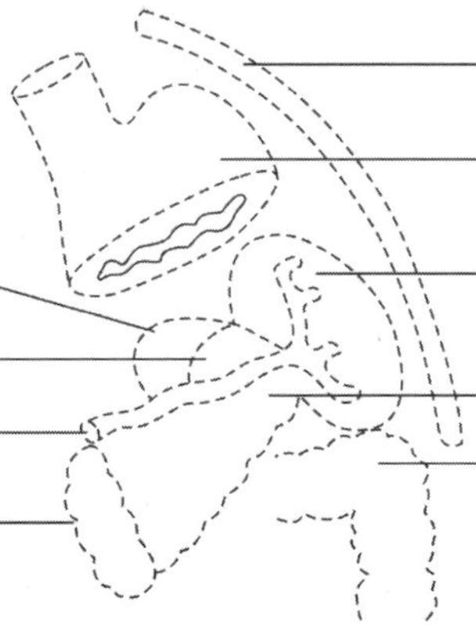

Figure 6.13: Spleen

KEY FEATURES

- Located in left hypochondrium between fundus of stomach and diaphragm, behind midaxillary line, directed downwards, forwards and laterally aligned along 9th–11th ribs
- Exhibits two ends—anterior and posterior, two borders—superior with 2–3 notches and inferior border, two surfaces—diaphragmatic and visceral related to stomach, left kidney, colon and tail of pancreas, two ligaments—gastrosplenic and lienorenal containing tail of pancreas, splenic artery
- Spleen is supported by phrenicocolic ligament.

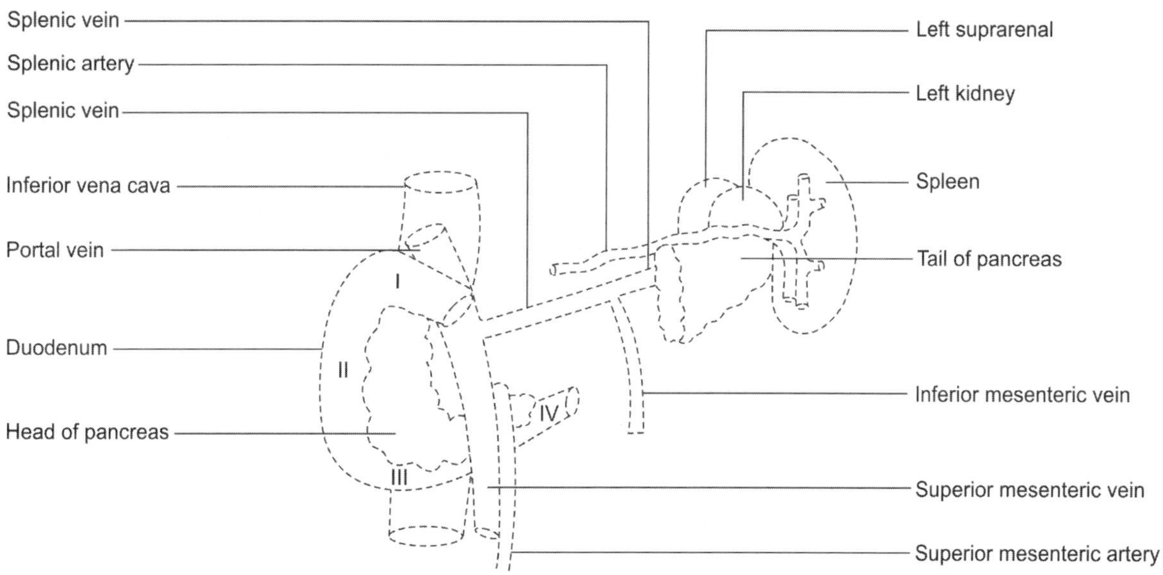

Figure 6.14: Pancreas

KEY FEATURES

- It is a mixed type of gland having exocrine component associated with gut and an endocrine component which is maximum in tail.
- It is divided into:
  - Head which lies in the concavity of duodenum and is flat anteroposteriorly
  - Neck which is narrow one inch long
  - Long body directed upwards and to the left and is triangular in shape
  - A tail which lies in lienorenal ligament with splenic vessels.
- Posteriorly (from right to left) related to:
  - Inferior vena cava
  - Common bile duct
  - Aorta
  - Left renal vein
  - Beginning of portal vein
  - Superior mesenteric vessels
  - Left kidney
  - Left suprarenal
  - Splenic vessels.
- Anteriorly (from right to left) related to:
  - Transverse colon
  - Root of transverse mesocolon
  - Pylorus
  - Lesser sac
  - Stomach
  - Duodenojejunal flexure
  - Jejunum
  - Left colic flexure

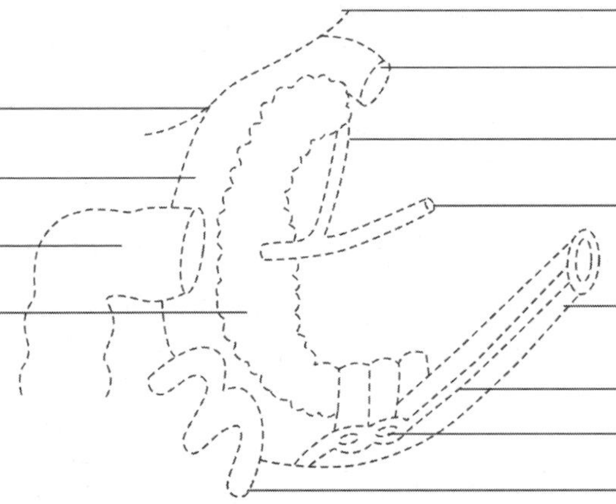

Figure 6.15: Duodenum—anterior relations

KEY FEATURES

- 1st part—quadrate lobe of liver
- 2nd part—right lobe of liver, transverse colon and jejunum
- 3rd part—superior mesenteric vessels, root of mesentery
- 4th part—transverse colon and its mesocolon.

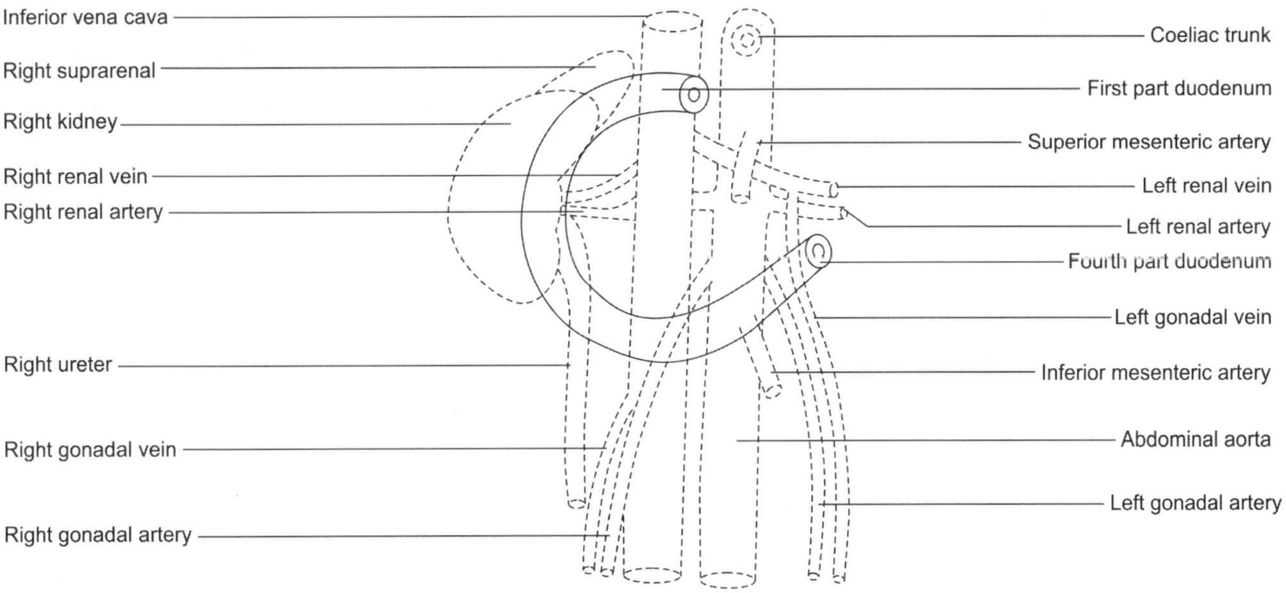

Figure 6.16: Duodenum—posterior relations

KEY FEATURES

- 1st part—portal vein, gastroduodenal artery, common bile duct
- 2nd part—right kidney, right renal vessels, right psoas major, inferior vena cava
- 3rd part—right psoas major, right ureter, inferior vena cava, abdominal aorta, gonadal vessels
- 4th part—left psoas major, left sympathetic chain, left gonadal vessels, left crus diaphragm, inferior mesenteric vessels.

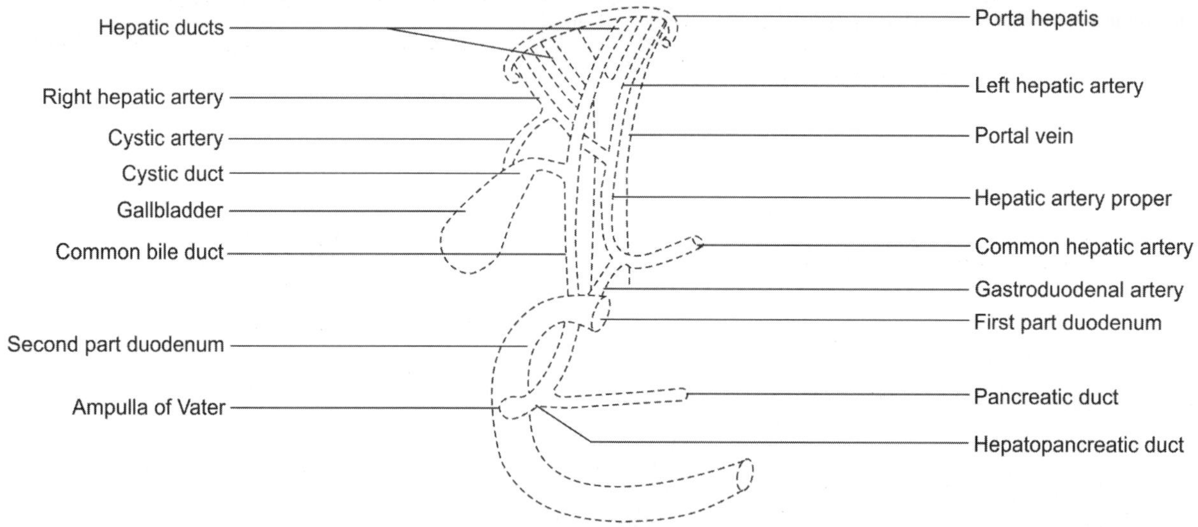

Figure 6.17: Extra biliary apparatus

KEY FEATURES

Comprises of:

- Right and left hepatic ducts which emerge from porta hepatis to form common hepatic duct 3 cm long and enters right free margin of lesser omentum
- Gallbladder 10 cm long, 3 cm wide, 30–50 mL capacity. It has fundus, body and neck which continues as cystic duct 3 cm long
- Common bile duct 7.5 cm long, formed by the union of cystic and common hepatic duct close to porta hepatis.

It lies to the right of hepatic artery, anterior to portal vein. These three structures run in right free margin of lesser omentum. It runs behind duodenum and unites with pancreatic duct to open on major duodenal papilla 8–10 cm distal to pylorus.

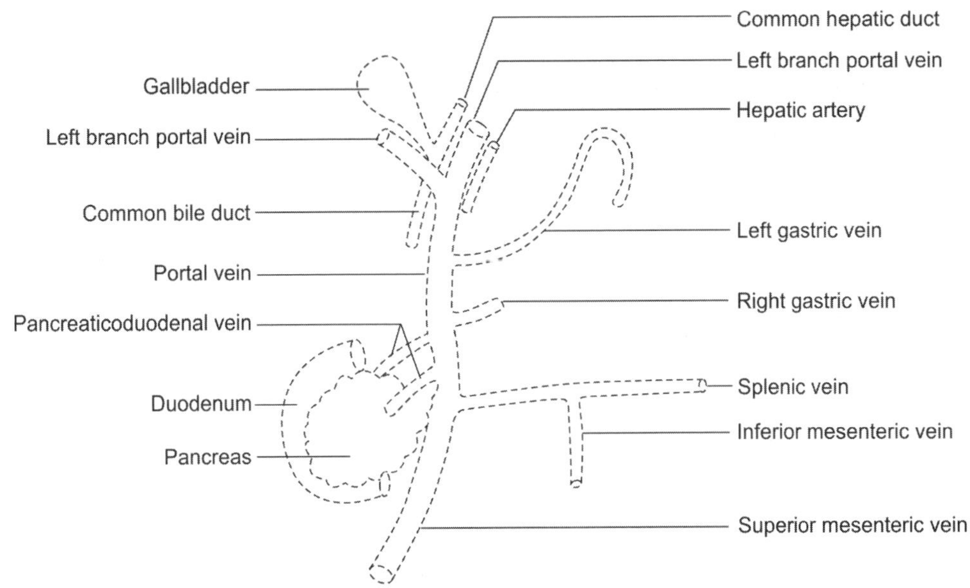

Figure 6.18: Portal vein

KEY FEATURES

- Portal vein provides 80% blood to liver
- It drains GIT, gallbladder, pancreas and spleen, it is 3" in length
- Formation: Behind the neck of pancreas by the union of splenic vein and superior mesenteric vein at the level of L2
- Superior mesenteric vein carries products of digestion and splenic vein carries products of RBC destruction to liver
- Course: Runs up and to the right behind first part of duodenum, then enters right free margin of lesser omentum accompanied by common bile duct and hepatic artery
- It enters liver, divides into right branch (short and wide) and left branch (long and narrow)
- Tributaries:
  - Splenic vein
  - Superior mesenteric vein
  - Cystic vein
  - Pancreaticoduodenal
  - Right and left gastric veins
  - Paraumbilical vein.

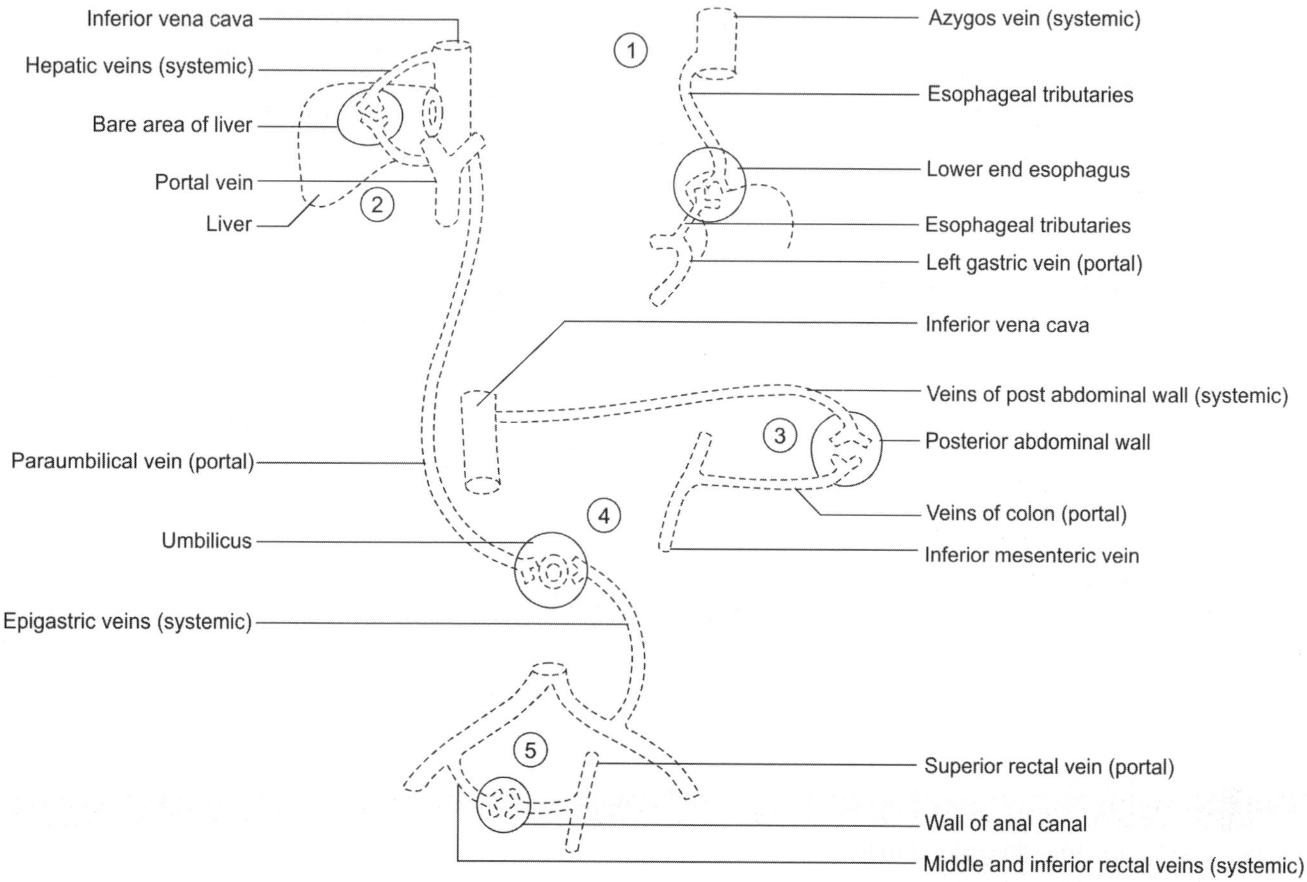

Figure 6.19: Portocaval anastomosis

KEY FEATURES

There are areas in body where systemic and portal venous systems anastomose. These sites are most commonly affected in portal hypertension.

S. No.	*Site*	*Systemic veins*	*Portal vein*	*Applied*
1	Lower end esophagus	Azygos	Left gastric	Esophageal varices, hematemesis
2	Bare area liver	Hepatic	Portal	—
3	Posterior abdominal wall	Veins of posterior abdominal wall	Veins of colon	
4	Umbilicus	Epigastric vein	Paraumbilical vein	Caput medusa
5	Wall of anal canal	Middle and inferior rectal veins	Superior rectal vein	Hemorrhoids

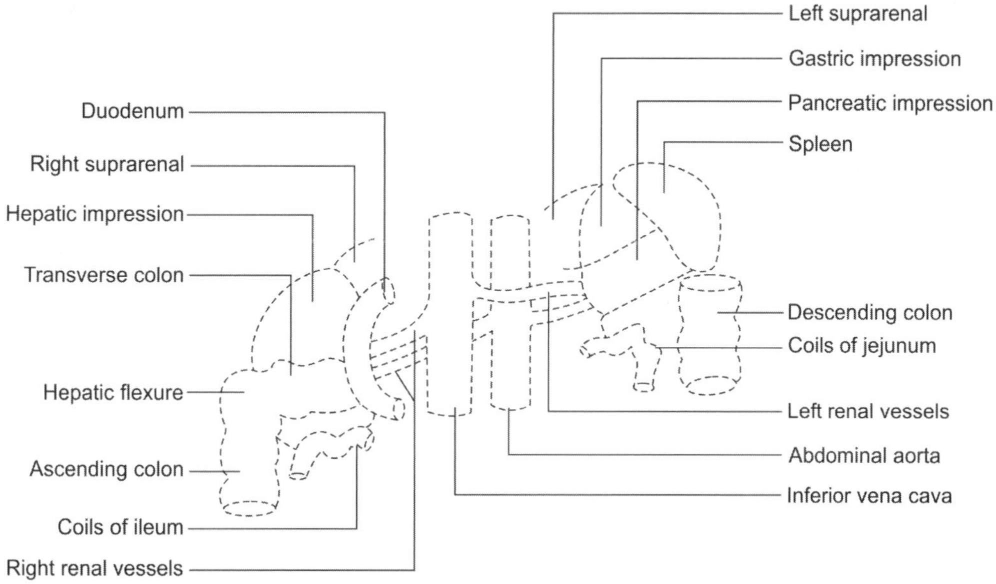

Figure 6.20: Kidneys—anterior relations

KEY FEATURES

- Right kidney: Above downwards
    - Right suprarenal
    - Right lobe liver
    - 2nd part duodenum
    - Hepatic flexure colon
    - Coils of ileum.
- Left kidney: Above downwards
    - Left suprarenal
    - Stomach
    - Spleen
    - Pancreas and splenic vessels
    - Jejunum
    - Descending colon.

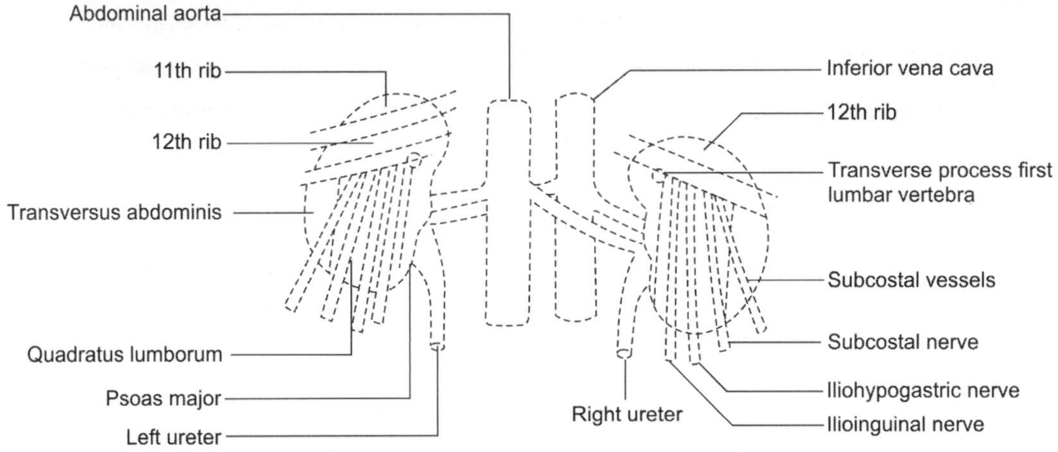

Figure 6.21: Kidneys—posterior relations

KEY FEATURES

Both the kidneys are related to:

- Diaphragm above the hilum.
- Below the hilum it is related to following structures in a mediolateral direction:
  - Psoas major
  - Quadratus lumborum
  - Ilioinguinal nerve
  - Iliohypogastric nerve
  - Subcostal nerve
  - Subcostal vessels
  - Transversus abdominis.

The only difference is that left kidney is related to 11th and 12th ribs being at higher level than right. The right kidney is related to 12th rib only.

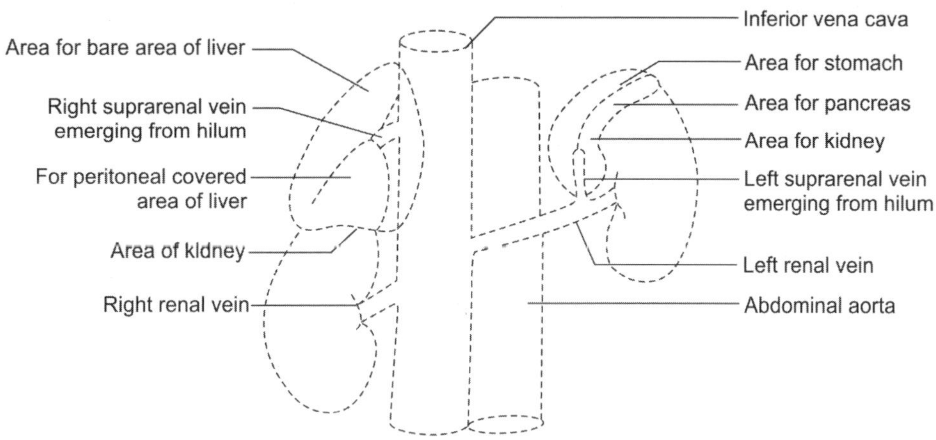

Figure 6.22: Suprarenals

KEY FEATURES

- Right suprarenal: Shape—like top hat, rests on upper pole of kidney, anterior surface divided into medial area related to inferior vena cava and a lateral area related to bare area of liver. Hilum near the upper end and the vein drains into inferior vena cava
- Left suprarenal: Shape—like bowler hat, inclines medially to reach hilum of kidney. Anterior surface divided into a superior area related to stomach and a inferior area related to pancreas. It is related to omental bursa. Hilum near the lower end and the vein drains into renal vein.

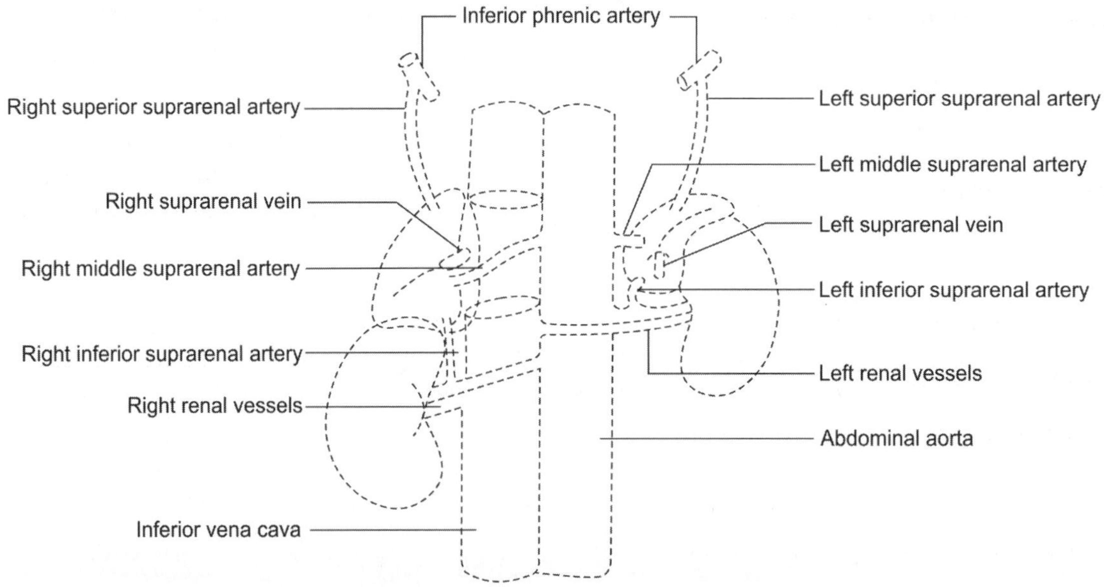

Figure 6.23: Suprarenals—blood supply

KEY FEATURES

- The suprarenal glands get their blood supply from three sources:
  i. Superior suprarenal artery—branch of inferior phrenic artery
  ii. Middle suprarenal artery—branch of abdominal aorta
  iii. Inferior suprarenal artery—branch of renal artery.
- Venous drainage:
  - Right vein drains into inferior vena cava
  - Left vein drains into left renal vein.

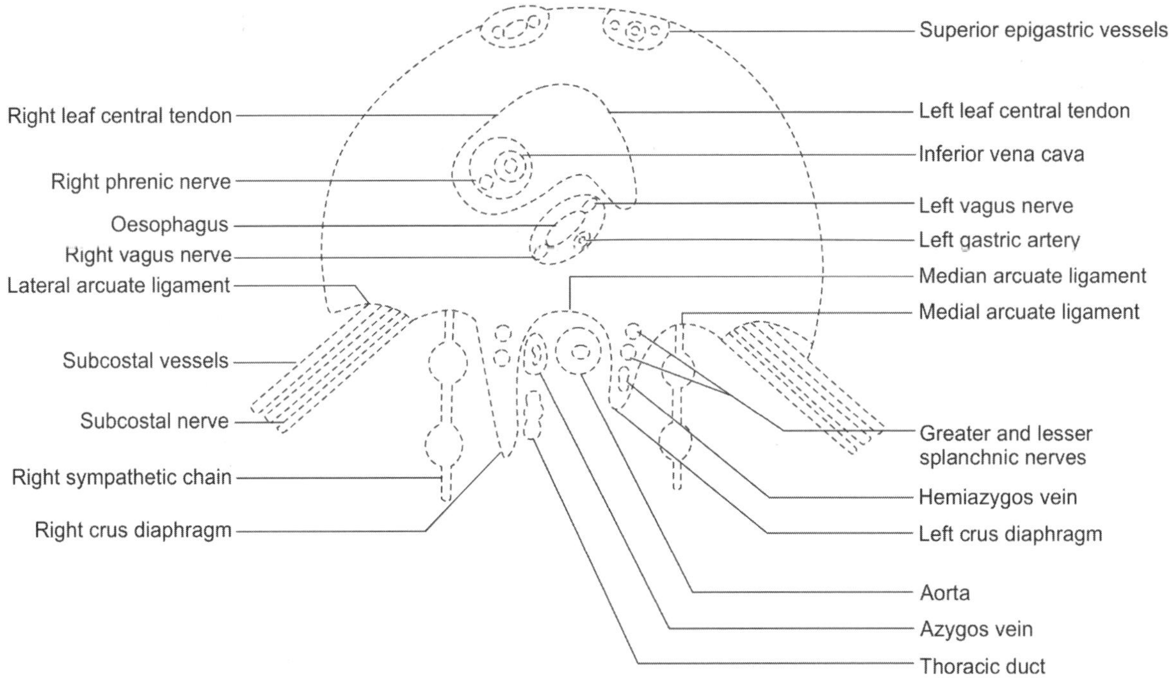

Figure 6.24: Apertures in diaphragm

KEY FEATURES

- Diaphragm is main muscle of respiration, has a peripheral muscular and a central tendinous part
- Central tendon trifoliate and fused with fibrous pericardium towards sternum
- The muscular part arises from sternum, ribs and vertebrae. The vertebral origin is by right and left crura. It presents lateral, medial and median arcuate ligaments
- Openings:
  - Aponeurotic for inferior vena cava and right phrenic nerve in right leaf of central tendon, quadrangular in shape, level T8.
  - Muscular for esophagus, right and left vagus, branches left gastric artery, oval in shape towards left, level T10.
  - Osseoaponeurotic for aorta, azygos vein and thoracic duct, level T12.

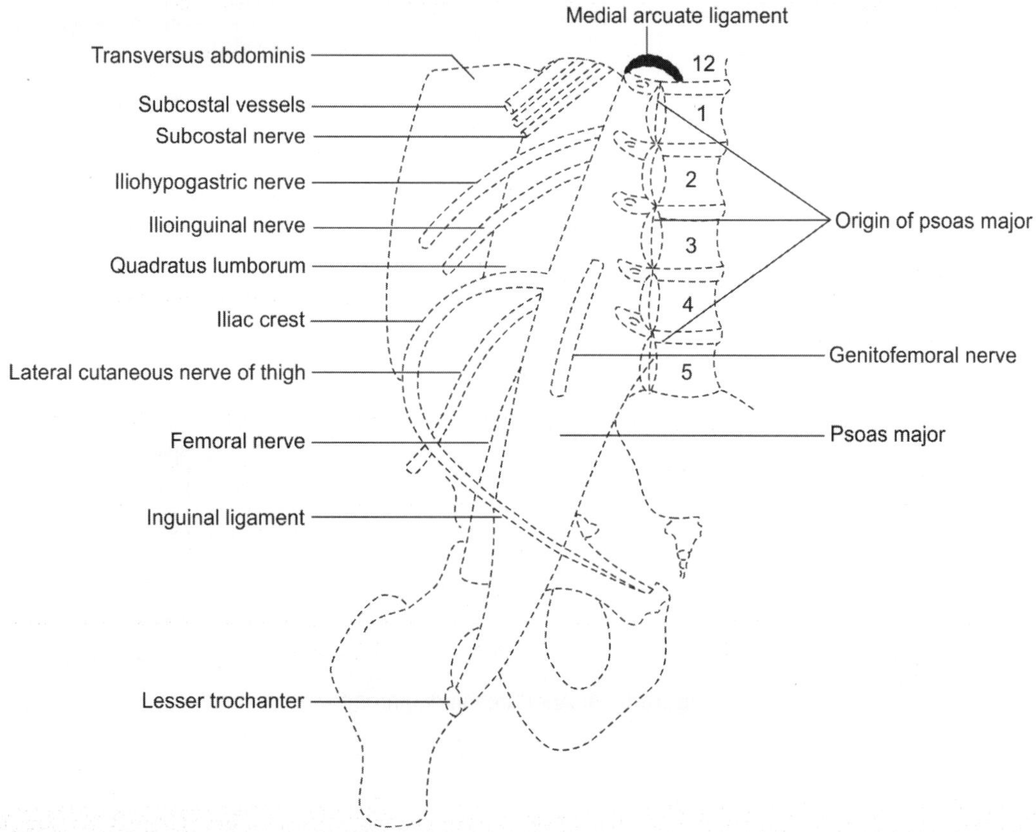

Figure 6.25: Posterior abdominal wall

KEY FEATURES

- Has three muscles from medial to lateral side: Psoas major, iliacus and quadratus lumborum
- Psoas major is related to six nerves laterally above downwards:
  - i. Subcostal
  - ii. Iliohypogastric
  - iii. Ilioinguinal
  - iv. Lateral cutaneous nerve of thigh
  - v. Femoral nerve. Genitofemoral nerve lies on its anterior surface.
  - vi. Obturator nerve emerges from medial side.
- Psoas arises from:
  - Intervertebral discs from T12 to L5.
  - Transverse processes from L1 to L5.
  - Four slips from tendinous arches. It is inserted along with iliacus on lesser trochanter of femur
- Lumbar plexus is formed within the substance of psoas
- It is covered by a sheath of fascia called psoas fascia
- In tuberculosis of lumbar vertebrae, the pus may spread along the emerging nerves and is called psoas abscess.
- Quadratus lumborum extends between 12th rib and iliac crest, it is enclosed by thoracolumbar fascia.

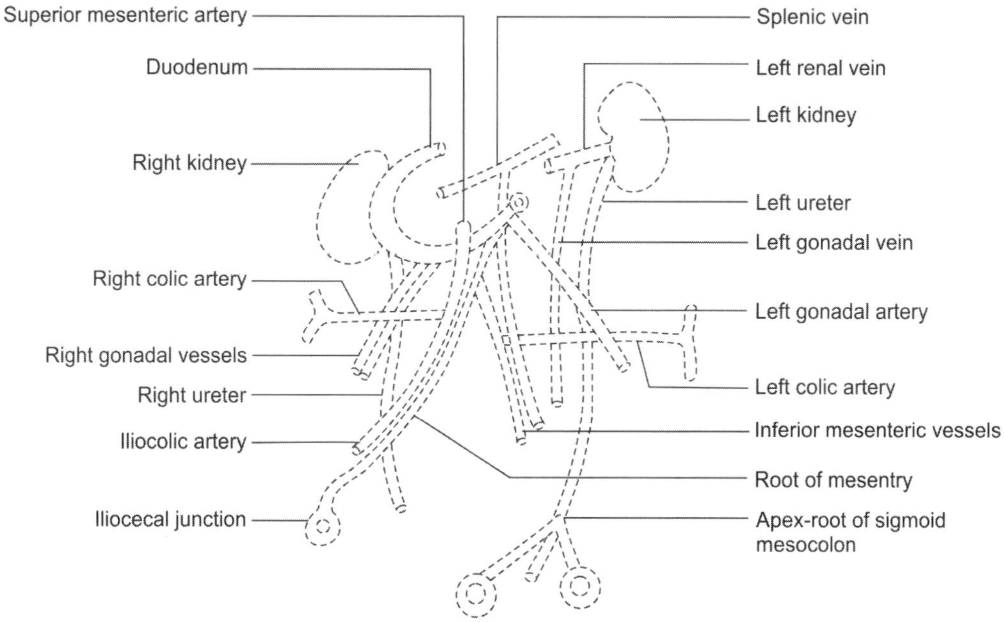

Figure 6.26: Ureter—Abdominal part in both sexes

KEY FEATURES

- Right ureter
  - Anteriorly related to 2nd part duodenum, gonadal vessels, root of mesentery, right colic and ileocolic vessels
  - Posteriorly related to right psoas and bifurcation of right common iliac artery
  - Medially related to inferior vena cava.
- Left ureter
  - Anteriorly related to left colic, sigmoidal and left gonadal vessels, sigmoid mesocolon
  - Posteriorly related to left psoas and bifurcation of left common iliac artery
  - Medially related to gonadal vessels and inferior mesenteric vein.

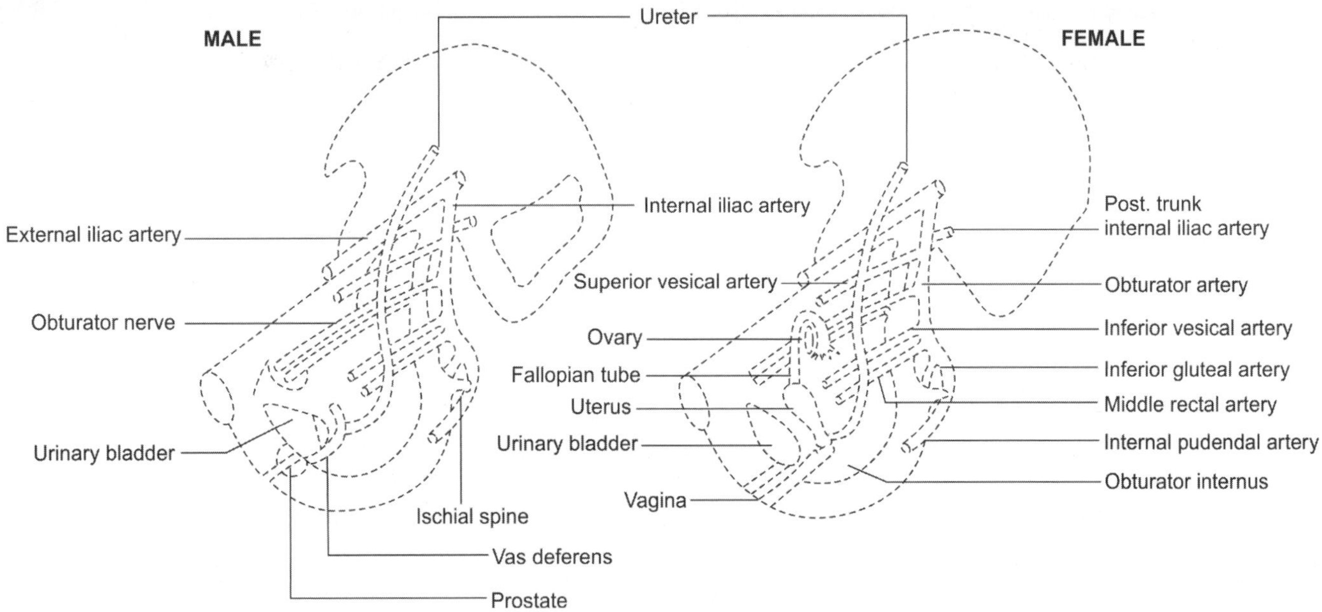

Figure 6.27: Ureter—pelvic part (male and female)

KEY FEATURES

In males

First part: Vertical, from pelvic brim to ischial spine.

- *Laterally* above downwards related to:
    - External iliac artery.
    - Superior vesical artery.
    - Obturator vessels and nerve.
    - Inferior vesical artery.
    - Middle rectal artery.
- *Medially*: Peritoneum

Second part: Oblique, runs forward and medially to reach urinary bladder.

- *Below and laterally*: Levator ani and fascia
- *Above and medially*: Covered by peritoneum, crossed by vas deferens
- *Below*: Seminal vesicle.

In females

First part: The course remains the same except that it forms the posterior boundary of ovarian fossa and crosses uterine and vaginal arteries.

Second part:

- *Above*: Broad ligament, uterine artery crosses ureter from lateral to medial side
- *Below*: (a) Mackenrodts ligament, (b) lateral fornix vagina, (c) levator ani
- *Medially*: Supravaginal part of cervix, anterior vaginal wall
- *Laterally*: Uterine artery before it crosses ureter.

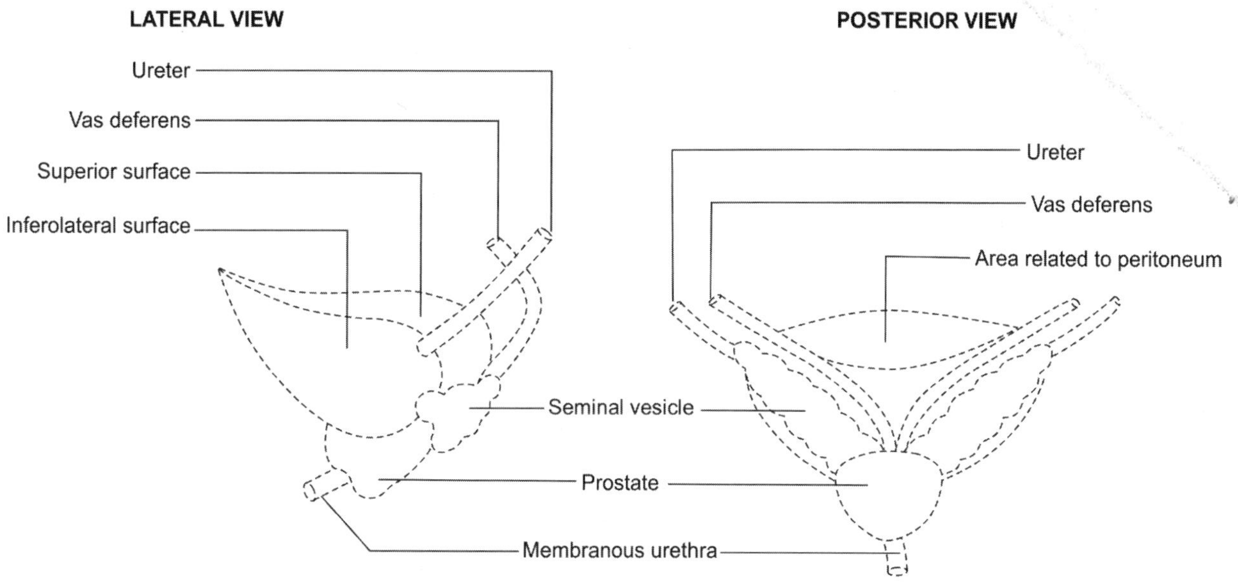

Figure 6.28: Urinary bladder—lateral view and posterior view

KEY FEATURES

- Tetrahedron when empty, ovoid when distended
- To the apex urachus is attached which raises median umbilical ligament
- Base: Triangular, directed posteroinferiorly. Ureters enter at superolateral angles.
  - In male, upper part forms anterior wall of rectovesical pouch and is related to peritoneum; lower part is not covered by peritoneum, it is related to vas deferens and seminal vesicle on each side
  - In females, it forms anterior wall of vesicouterine pouch.
- Inferolateral surface: Not related to peritoneum
- Superior surface:
  - In males—covered by peritoneum, related to ileum
  - In females—no peritoneum near posterior border.

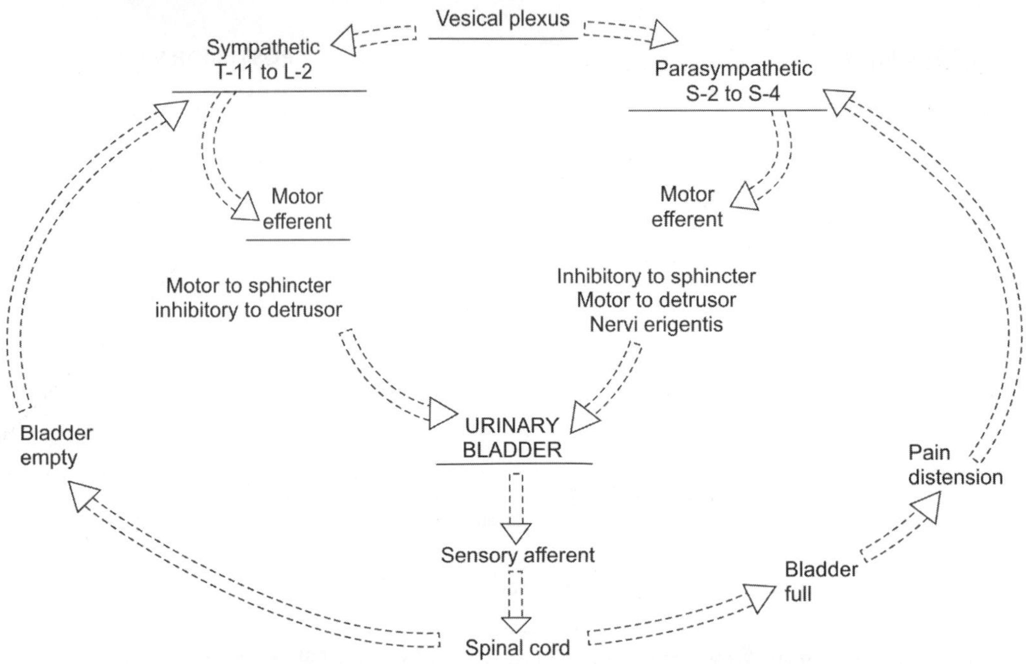

Figure 6.29: Urinary bladder—nerve supply

KEY FEATURES

- The vesical plexus derived from inferior hypogastric plexus contains both parasympathetic and sympathetic fibers
- The pathway depends whether urinary bladder is full or empty and is mediated through spinal cord
- In bladder distension parasympathetic (S2–S4) through nervi erigentis causes evacuation of bladder
- Once bladder is emptied, the sympathetic (T11–L2) system causes refilling of bladder by closing the sphincter.

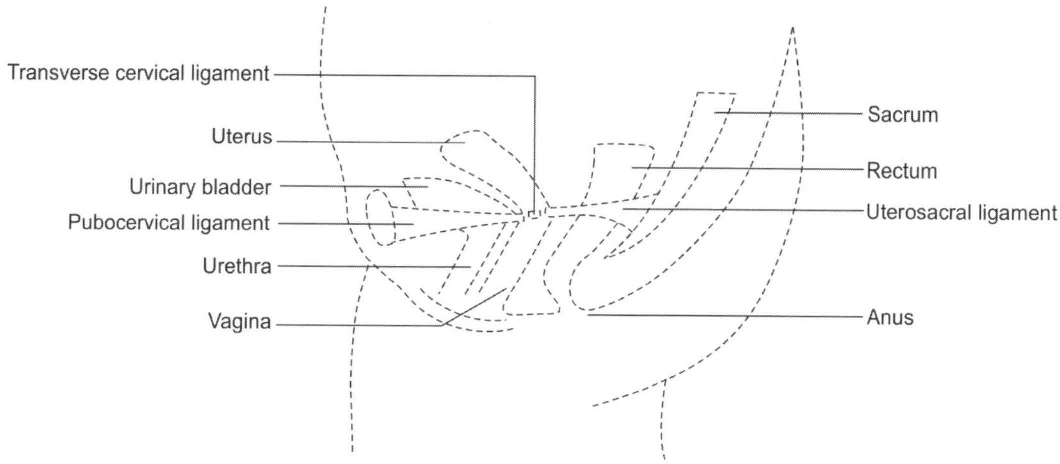

Figure 6.30: Supports of uterus—lateral view

KEY FEATURES

➡ Primary supports:

- Muscular
  - Pelvic diaphragm
  - Perineal body
  - Urogenital diaphragm.
- Fibromuscular
  - Transverse cervical
  - Pubocervical
  - Uterosacral
  - Round ligaments.
- Visceral
  - Urinary bladder
  - Vagina
  - Uterine axis.

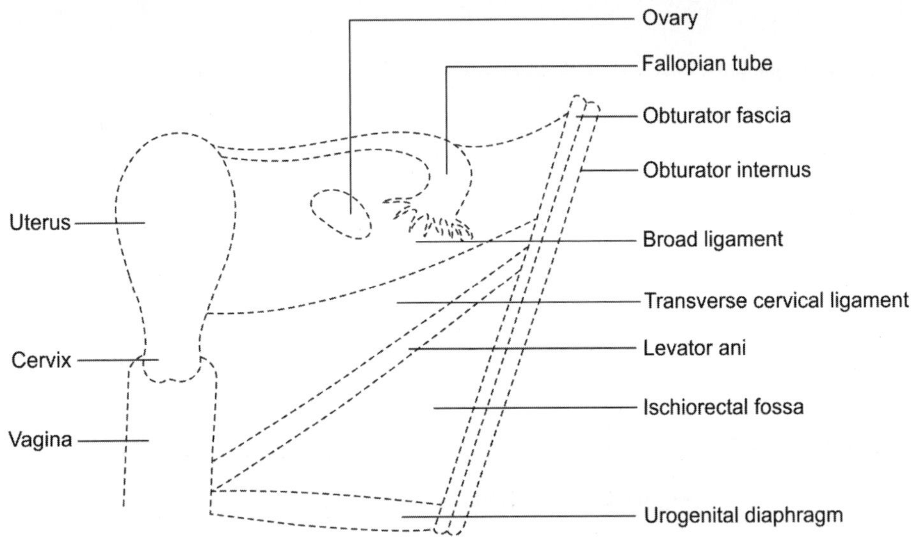

Figure 6.31: Supports of uterus—anterior view

KEY FEATURES

Secondary supports: They are basically folds of peritoneum:

- Broad ligament of uterus.
- Uterovesical fold.
- Rectovaginal fold.

Transverse cervical ligament is important and is called cardinal ligament. It is condensed pelvic fascia around uterine vessels

Extent: From cervix and upper vagina to lateral pelvic wall

Function: Prevents downward displacement of uterus.

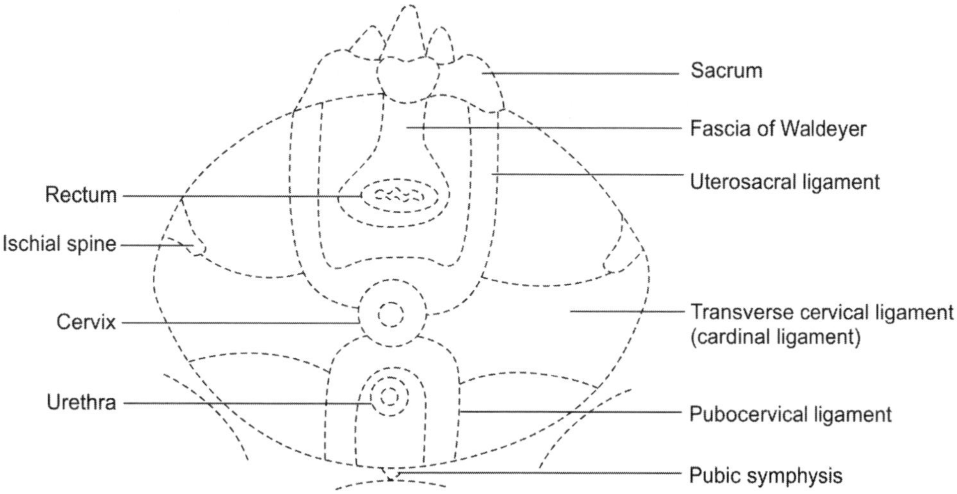

Figure 6.32: Supports of uterus—superior view

KEY FEATURES

- Shows fibromuscular supports of uterus
- Pubocervical ligament: Runs between pubis and cervix of uterus on either side of urethra
- Uterosacral ligament: Runs between cervix and S2-3 vertebrae on either side of rectum. It forms lateral boundary of rectouterine pouch.
- Function:
  - Pulls cervix backwards.
  - Counteracts the pull of round ligament.
  - Maintains antiflexed and antiverted position of uterus.

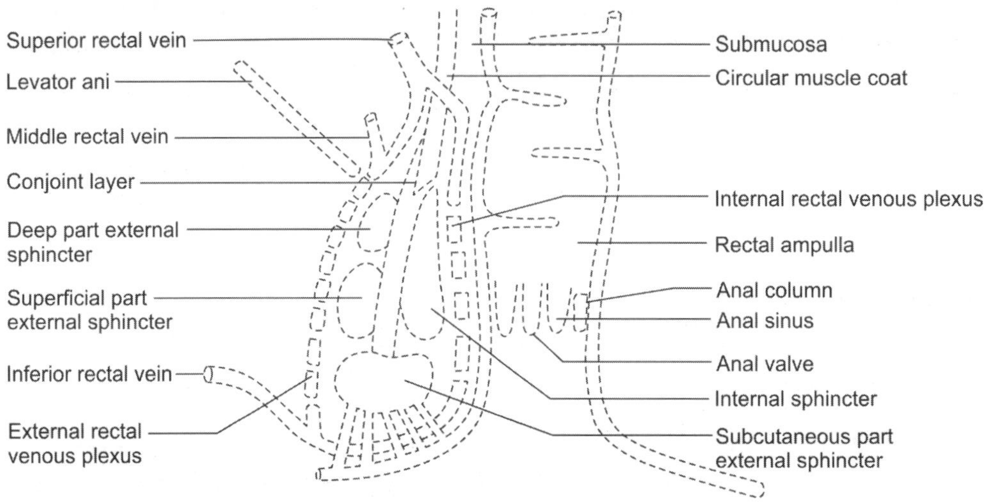

Figure 6.33: Rectum and anal canal

KEY FEATURES

- Rectum:
  - 12 cm long, 4 cm wide, lower part dilated called ampulla
  - Upper 1/3rd covered by peritoneum anteriorly and laterally
  - Middle 1/3rd covered by peritoneum anteriorly only
  - Lower 1/3rd not related to peritoneum
  - It forms rectovesical/rectouterine pouch
  - Arterial supply: Superior rectal (1) continuation of inferior mesenteric. Middle rectal (2) branch of anterior division of internal iliac. Inferior rectal (2) branch of internal pudendal.
- Anal canal:
  - Anterior wall shorter than posterior wall, sphincter ani muscle keeps the canal closed. Length 38 mm.
  - Anal canal is guarded by anal sphincters: (a) internal, (b) external
  - The external anal sphincter has (a) subcutaneous part, (b) superficial part, (c) deep part
  - Anteriorly—perineal body. Posteriorly—anococcygeal raphe. On sides ischiorectal fossa.
  - Internally—
    - Upper 15 mm lies above pectinate line, has 6–10 anal columns which contain veins. The columns are united by anal valves of Ball indicated by wavy pectinate line. These valves have anal sinus.
    - Middle 15 mm between pectinate and line of Hilton called area of pectin.
    - Lower 8 mm lined by true skin below the line of Hilton.
  - The rectal veins arise from internal rectal venous plexus to form:
    - Superior rectal vein which drains into portal vein through inferior mesenteric vein.
    - Middle rectal veins drain into internal iliac veins.
    - Inferior rectal veins run across ischiorectal fossa and drain into internal pudendal vein.

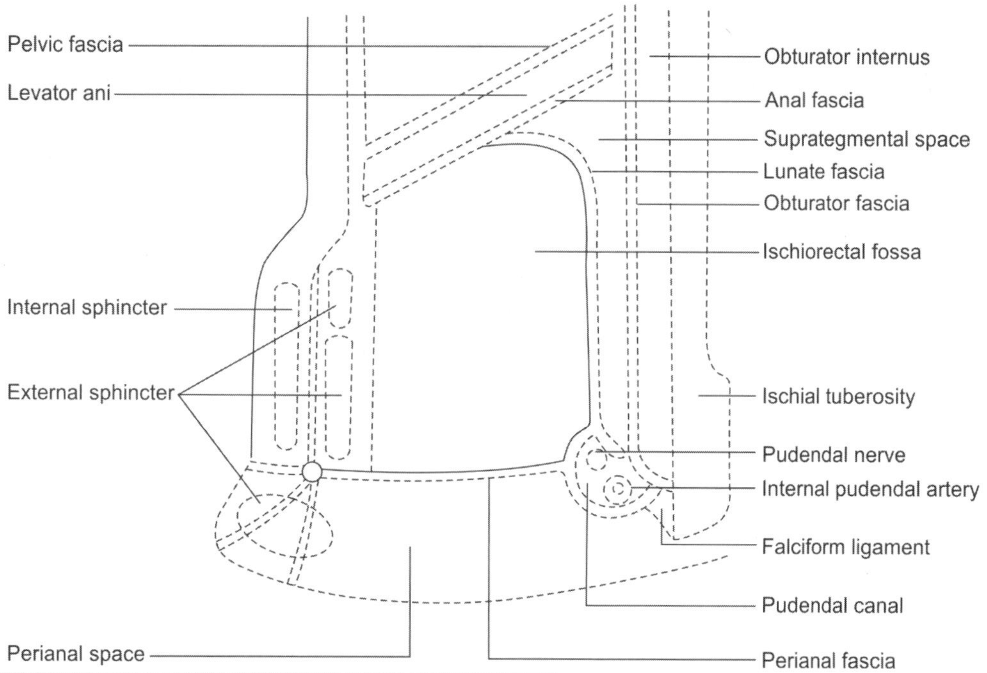

Figure 6.34: Ischiorectal fossa—coronal section

KEY FEATURES

- It is wedge-shaped, fat filled space on each side of anal canal, below pelvic diaphragm, continuous with each other
- Function: Dilatation of anal canal
- Base—skin; apex—upwards and laterally; lateral wall—fascia covering obturator internus, ischial tuberosity and pudendal canal; medially—fascia covering levator ani, external anal sphincter; posteriorly—sacrotuberous ligament, gluteus maximus; anteriorly—perineal membrane; floor—perianal skin; roof—meeting of medial and lateral walls
- Spaces: (a) suprategmental, (b) ischiorectal, (c) perianal
- Contents:
  - Internal pudendal vessels and nerve.
  - Inferior rectal vessels and nerve.
  - Posterior scrotal/labial vessels and nerve.
  - Perineal branch of S4.

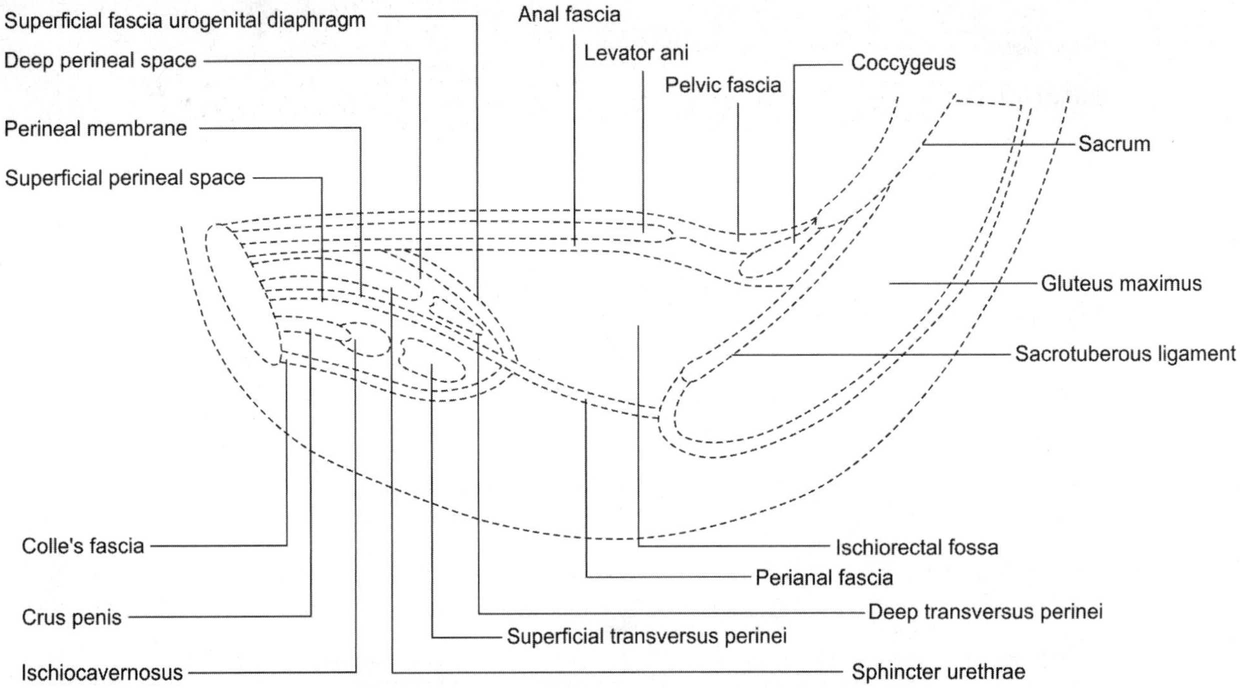

Figure 6.35: Perineal pouches—parasagittal section

KEY FEATURES

- There are two perineal pouches which lie in the gap between pubic arch
- These pouches are separated by perineal membrane (inferior fascia of urogenital diaphragm)
- Perineal membrane: Laterally—ischiopubic rami. Anteriorly forms transverse perineal ligament and continues with superior fascia of urogenital diaphragm. Posteriorly—fixes perineal body and splits into two layers: (a) Upper layer continues with superior fascia of urogenital diaphragm, (b) Lower layer continues with Colles fascia
- Superior perineal pouch is bounded by: Perineal membrane above, Colle's fascia below, ischiopubic rami on sides. It is closed posteriorly but open anteriorly and continues with superficial inguinal space. Contents: (1) Ischiocavernosus, (2) Crus penis, (3) Superficial transversus perinei muscle
- Deep perineal pouch is bounded by: Superior fascia of urogenital diaphragm above, perineal membrane below, ischiopubic rami on sides. It is closed both posteriorly and anteriorly.

Contents: (1) Sphincter urethrae (2) Deep transversus perinei muscle

- These two muscles constitute urogenital diaphragm.

Function: (1) Supports bladder and prostate, (2) Constricts vagina, (3) Fixes perineal body, (4) Expels last drop of urine.